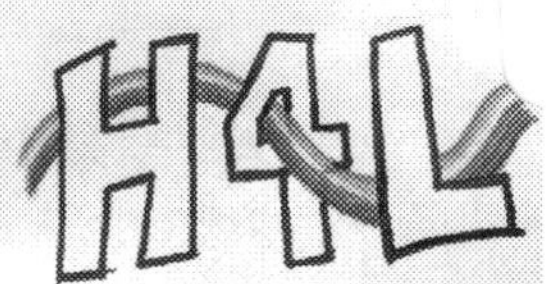

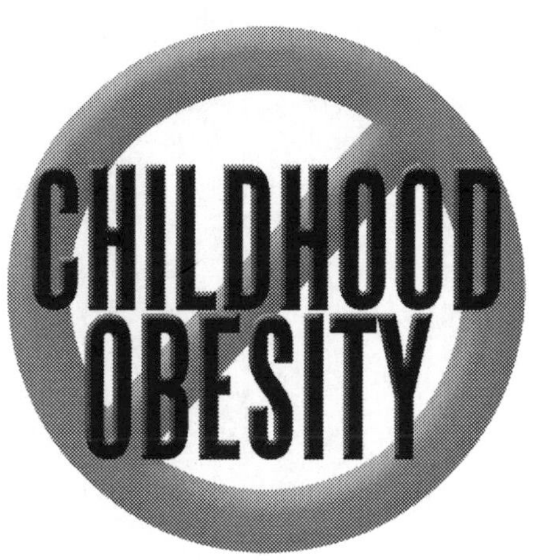

MY HEALTHY FOR LIFE JOURNAL

Dr. Olga Vaca Durr

A journal to use in conjunction with …

It's **NOT** about

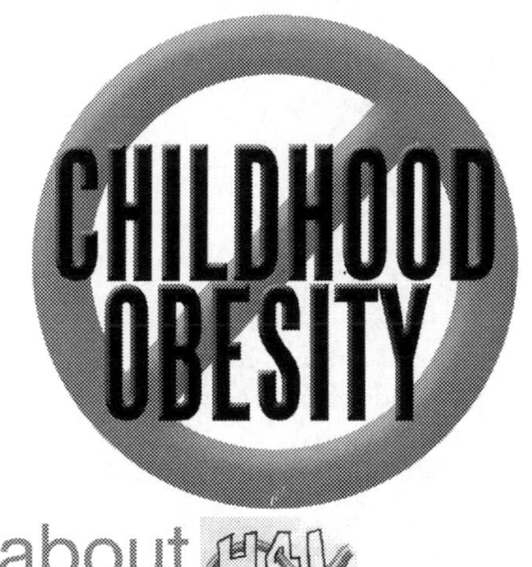

It **IS** about H4L

MY HEALTHY FOR LIFE JOURNAL

Dr. Olga Vaca Durr

Inspiring Voices®
A Service of Guideposts

Inspiring Voices books may be ordered through booksellers or by contacting:

Inspiring Voices
1663 Liberty Drive
Bloomington, IN 47403
www.inspiringvoices.com
1-(866) 697-5313

ISBN: 978-1-4624-0481-0 (sc)
ISBN: 978-1-4624-0482-7 (e)

Library of Congress Control Number: 2012923962

Printed in the United States of America

Inspiring Voices rev. date:1/3/2013

To Naomi Arriaga Vaca:

Thanks, Momma, for believing I could do things

I never thought I could even reach!

To George E. Peyrot Jr.:

Thanks, George, for showing me running is not all that bad!

It's about being healthy for life!

—H4L

Table of Contents

Preface

As I completed my book, *It's Not about Childhood Obesity, It Is about Being Healthy for Life*, I realized it would be much easier for people to get started on their new healthy for life lifestyles if they had the proper tools. So I got all my tools and resources together—all the information I had written—and started on this journal.

I hope you are able to incorporate this journal into your everyday life to help you stay accountable to the most important person in your life. Always remember, it's not about size or shape and it's not about skinny or fluffy; it *is* about being healthy!

As you learn more about this healthy for life lifestyle and begin to balance your scale, I hope you are able to wean yourself off the journal at times. However, when you realize the scale is tipping, recognize that the journal is sitting around waiting to help out.

I know for me, even after all these years of attempting to live healthy for life, I still have my journal sitting around waiting to help me out. Sometimes I need my journal before and around the holidays, when I'm visiting family, during moves, or when I notice my scale is going wild. After you get accustomed to the healthy for life lifestyle, consider the journal as more of a support system than just a journal.

Acknowledgments

I would like to express my sincere appreciation and thanks to my husband, children, Daddy, and family members who encouraged my efforts to make this book a reality. Thank you for the comments, concerns, listening when I needed help, and your support.

Thank you to Dr. J. Austin Vasek for helping me complete my first enormous task, which was my initial research. Also, thank you to Dr. Randy Baca, Dr. Genie Jhnigoor, and Dr. Patti D. Ward for joining me as we completed that task.

Thanks to my niece, Elise Peyrot, (affectionately known as Ms. P by her students) for lending a creative, talented hand at various tasks throughout this journal. Love you Mija!

Also, thank you to Jack Pike for his photography. Mr. Pike is a true American hero. Check him out on Facebook at Jack T. F. Pike.

Disclaimer

The information provided in *It's Not about Childhood Obesity*; It Is about *Being Healthy for Life!* and *My Healthy for Life Journal* is intended as a general tool and reference for readers. The author is not rendering professional medical services, and the content is made available with this understanding. Although the author made every effort to provide current and accurate information, readers should be aware that the author accepts no responsibility for the accuracy and completeness of the material in this book and recommends consulting a doctor before making any major dietary or physical changes. Although the purpose of this book is to educate, the author shall have neither liability nor responsibility to any person or entity with respect to any loss or damage caused or suspected to be caused, either directly or indirectly, by the information contained in this book.

Introduction

This journal includes six sections, each spanning three months and includes space to write your goals, measurements, and add a picture if you would like. Each section also includes room to write or update your recommended daily allowance and keep track of your daily caloric intake and physical activity.

After each three-month period, you can update your goals and measurements, add a new picture, and determine if any changes need to be made in your recommended daily allowance according to your current weight and physical activity. As your weight and physical activity change, your recommended daily allowance may change some as well.

I know for me there were times when I was discouraged because no matter how hard I was working, I did not appear to be getting to a healthier weight. Then I realized my measurements were showing that I was actually making some improvements. Although I was not losing weight, I was building muscle and losing inches.

The journal is arranged in three-month sections. Therefore, you can start wherever is best for you. Since the dates are not written already, you are not locked into a certain period, which makes it nice if you do not start this journal on January 1. Therefore, make sure to write the dates down as you go. I have added two years of calendars in the front of the journal for your convenience.

In each section, there is room to add and update your goals. When I was in college, I learned the ABCs, and they didn't just pertain to the alphabet. I learned the ABCs of writing lesson plans, the ABCs of writing behavior goals, and the ABCs of writing IEPs (individual education plans), and I soon realized the ABCs could pertain to just about anything. In this instance, when writing goals in your *Healthy for Life Journal,* keep these ABCs in mind:

A: Audience—who do you expect to do something different? (Hint: Since these goals are for you, *you* are the target audience.)

B: Behavior—what behavior changes are you expecting to see?

C: Condition or circumstances—under what circumstances or condition will changes occur, or by when should results occur?

D: Degree—to what degree will change occur?

E: Evidence—what evidence will you use to measure changes that have occurred? Since you will be writing your goals down and keeping a physical activity log, your evidence will be listed in one of these two spots.

When incorporating the ABCs of writing goals in your *Healthy for Life Journal,* a goal may look like this: I (audience) will walk (behavior) thirty minutes per day (degree), four days per week (condition). The evidence will show in my physical activity log.

As for measurements, take them from the following places on your body, as well as writing down your weight and BMI:

- Your neck
- Your chest
- Your bicep
- Your waist
- Your hips
- Your thighs

Your BMI can be obtained from the following website: *http://apps.nccd.cdc.gov/dnpabmi/)*

Pictures are a great way to document and show progress. They can also get you excited about positive results. They personally keep me motivated to stay the course.

Finally, each section has room for you to document and keep track of your daily caloric intake and physical activity. There is room to write down what your recommended daily allowance is according to the website: www.choosemyplate.gov. I hope this journal allows you not only to be healthy for life but also to enjoy the benefits it provides not only you but your family and those around you as well.

As you start your healthy for life journey, I have a few things I want you to keep in mind. The following are just a few additional pointers to help you as you get started.

- Don't try to incorporate everything the first week.
- Start off with small, manageable goals.
- Set goals, schedules, and deadlines.
- Add nutritious food whenever you can.
- Eat breakfast every morning.
- Limit red meat consumption.
- Try some fish, chicken, or turkey.
- Make a game out of exercising.
- Add a little competition.
- Make a weekly menu.
- Drink some milk.
- *Celebrate your achievements, and stay balanced.*

2013 Calendar

January							February							March						
S	M	T	W	T	F	S	S	M	T	W	T	F	S	S	M	T	W	T	F	S
		1	2	3	4	5						1	2						1	2
6	7	8	9	10	11	12	3	4	5	6	7	8	9	3	4	5	6	7	8	9
13	14	15	16	17	18	19	10	11	12	13	14	15	16	10	11	12	13	14	15	16
20	21	22	23	24	25	26	17	18	19	20	21	22	23	17	18	19	20	21	22	23
27	28	29	30	31			24	25	26	27	28			24/31	25	26	27	28	29	30

April							May							June						
S	M	T	W	T	F	S	S	M	T	W	T	F	S	S	M	T	W	T	F	S
	1	2	3	4	5	6				1	2	3	4							1
7	8	9	10	11	12	13	5	6	7	8	9	10	11	2	3	4	5	6	7	8
14	15	16	17	18	19	20	12	13	14	15	16	17	18	9	10	11	12	13	14	15
21	22	23	24	25	26	27	19	20	21	22	23	24	25	16	17	18	19	20	21	22
28	29	30					26	27	28	29	30	31		23	24	25	26	27	28	29

July							August							September						
S	M	T	W	T	F	S	S	M	T	W	T	F	S	S	M	T	W	T	F	S
	1	2	3	4	5	6					1	2	3	1	2	3	4	5	6	7
7	8	9	10	11	12	13	4	5	6	7	8	9	10	8	9	10	11	12	13	14
14	15	16	17	18	19	20	11	12	13	14	15	16	17	15	16	17	18	19	20	21
21	22	23	24	25	26	27	18	19	20	21	22	23	24	22	23	24	25	26	27	28
28	29	30	31				25	26	27	28	29	30	31	29	30					

October							November							December						
S	M	T	W	T	F	S	S	M	T	W	T	F	S	S	M	T	W	T	F	S
		1	2	3	4	5						1	2	1	2	3	4	5	6	7
6	7	8	9	10	11	12	3	4	5	6	7	8	9	8	9	10	11	12	13	14
13	14	15	16	17	18	19	10	11	12	13	14	15	16	15	16	17	18	19	20	21
20	21	22	23	24	25	26	17	18	19	20	21	22	23	22	23	24	25	26	27	28
27	28	29	30	31			24	25	26	27	28	29	30	29	30	31				

2014 Calendar

January							February							March						
S	M	T	W	T	F	S	S	M	T	W	T	F	S	S	M	T	W	T	F	S
			1	2	3	4							1							1
5	6	7	8	9	10	11	2	3	4	5	6	7	8	2	3	4	5	6	7	8
12	13	14	15	16	17	18	9	10	11	12	13	14	15	9	10	11	12	13	14	15
19	20	21	22	23	24	25	16	17	18	19	20	21	22	16	17	18	19	20	21	22
26	27	28	29	30	31		23	24	25	26	27	28		23	24	25	26	27	28	29
														30	31					

April							May							June						
S	M	T	W	T	F	S	S	M	T	W	T	F	S	S	M	T	W	T	F	S
		1	2	3	4	5					1	2	3	1	2	3	4	5	6	7
6	7	8	9	10	11	12	4	5	6	7	8	9	10	8	9	10	11	12	13	14
13	14	15	16	17	18	19	11	12	13	14	15	16	17	15	16	17	18	19	20	21
20	21	22	23	24	25	26	18	19	20	21	22	23	24	22	23	24	25	26	27	28
27	28	29	30				25	26	27	28	29	30	31	29	30					

July							August							September						
S	M	T	W	T	F	S	S	M	T	W	T	F	S	S	M	T	W	T	F	S
		1	2	3	4	5						1	2		1	2	3	4	5	6
6	7	8	9	10	11	12	3	4	5	6	7	8	9	7	8	9	10	11	12	13
13	14	15	16	17	18	19	10	11	12	13	14	15	16	14	15	16	17	18	19	20
20	21	22	23	24	25	26	17	18	19	20	21	22	23	21	22	23	24	25	26	27
27	28	29	30	31			24	25	26	27	28	29	30	28	29	30				
							31													

October							November							December						
S	M	T	W	T	F	S	S	M	T	W	T	F	S	S	M	T	W	T	F	S
			1	2	3	4							1		1	2	3	4	5	6
5	6	7	8	9	10	11	2	3	4	5	6	7	8	7	8	9	10	11	12	13
12	13	14	15	16	17	18	9	10	11	12	13	14	15	14	15	16	17	18	19	20
19	20	21	22	23	24	25	16	17	18	19	20	21	22	21	22	23	24	25	26	27
26	27	28	29	30	31		23	24	25	26	27	28	29	28	29	30	31			

Where to Take Measurements (Pic)

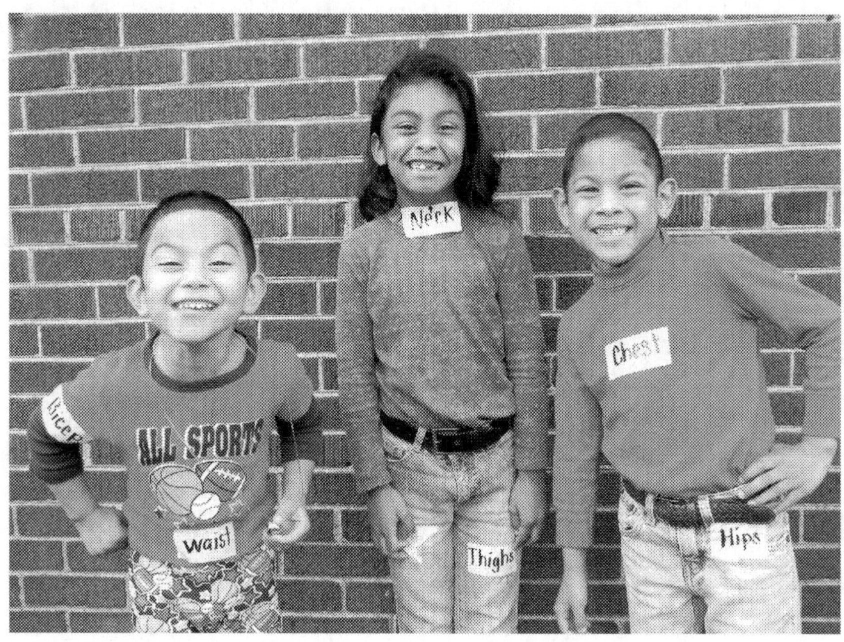

Section 1

Dates

_______ to _______

This is your initial or baseline section on your journey to being healthy for life.

My suggestion is to get a week of baseline data first and then write three to five goals. (You may have done this already.) When writing your goals, try to have at least one related to physical activity and one related to caloric intake. Keep in mind, you should take small steps!

Initial Goals on Your Healthy for Life Journey

Check the box when a goal is achieved, and write the date it was achieved on the line next to the box. Write a goal next to the number, keeping in mind the ABCs.

Date Achieved — Goal

☐______ 1. ________________________________

☐______ 2. ________________________________

☐______ 3. ________________________________

☐______ 4. ________________________________

Initial Measurement of *You* on Your Healthy for Life Journey

Date: ____________________

Location	Measurement
Neck	
Chest	
Bicep	
Waist	
Hips	
Thighs	
Weight	
BMI	

Initial Picture of *You* on Your Healthy for Life Journey

Date: ______________________

The Key to Healthy Weight

The key to healthy weight is the balance between caloric intake and physical activity.

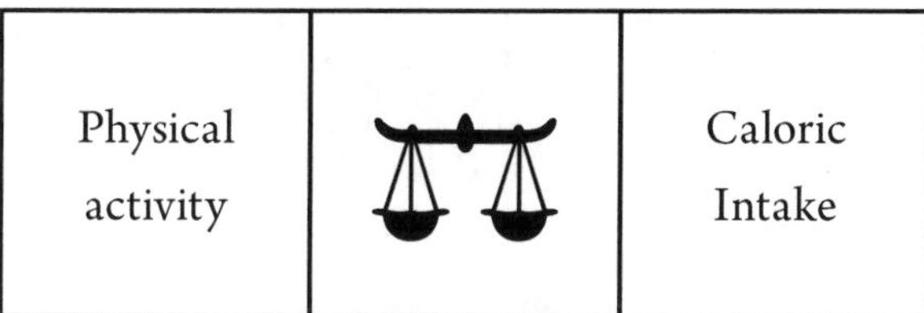

Secret to Weight Loss ...

Honesty!

Be completely honest with yourself about everything regarding your caloric intake and your physical activity!

Recommended Daily Allowance

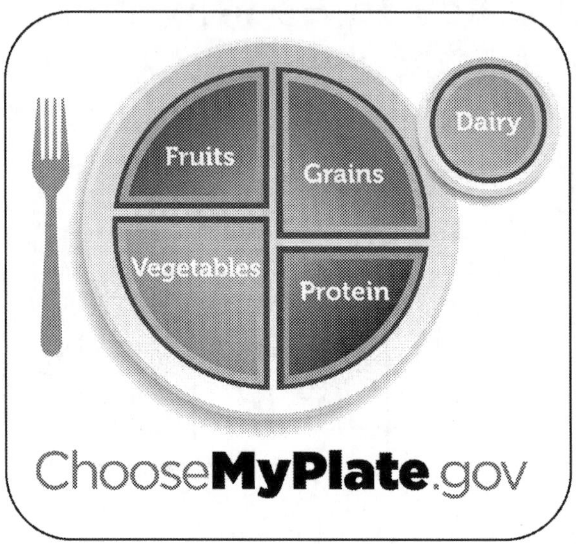

Go to the following website: www.choosemyplate.gov to find out what your recommend daily allowance (RDA), or caloric intake, should include and write it down.

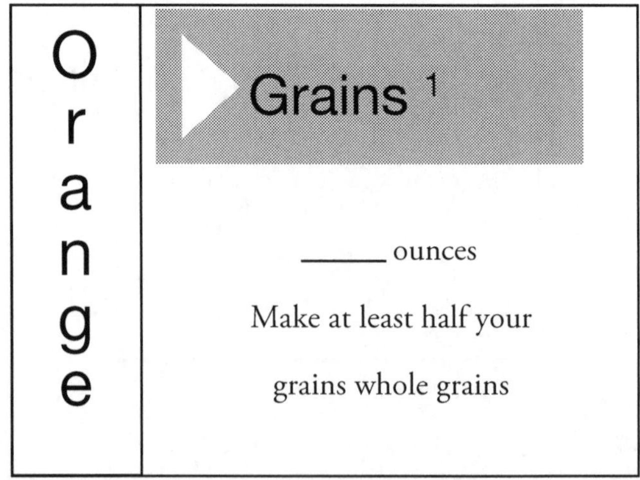

Green	**Vegetables** [2] _____ cups Try to include: dark green, red, & orange; beans & peas, starchy, & other veggies
Red	**Fruits** _____ cups Select fresh, frozen, canned, & dried fruit more often than juie
Blue	**Dairy** _____ cups Include fat-free and low-fat dairy foods every day

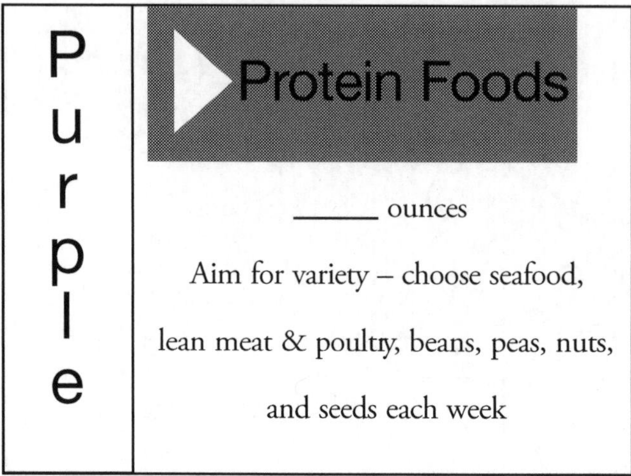

In a few months, go back to see if this has changed. As you begin to include more physical activity and your weight decreases to a healthier weight, these numbers may change.

Weekly Calorie Intake

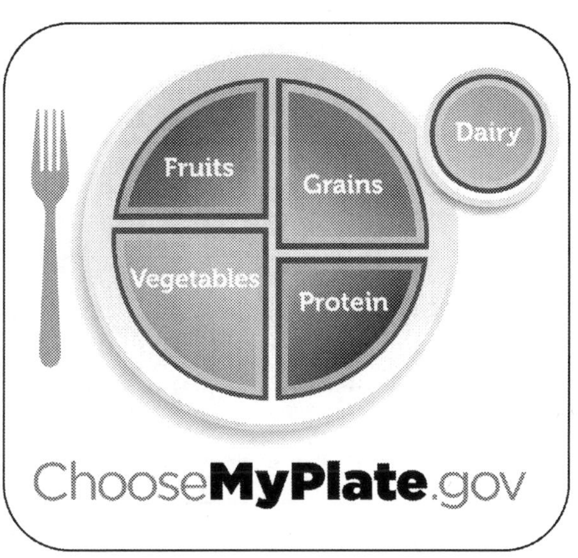

Weekly include:

Dark Green Vegetables: ______ cups

Orange Vegetables: ______ cups

Dry Beans & Peas: ______ cups

Starchy Vegetables: ______ cups

Other Vegetables: ______ cups

New Foods I will try this quarter

Grains: ______________________

____

____

Vegetables: ______________________

____

____

Fruits: ______________________

____

____

Dairy: ______________________

____

____

Protein: ______________________

____

____

How to use your weekly caloric intake log:

Write the date under the day of the week.

8: cross off an 8 for each eight ounces of water you drink each day.

F: cross off an F for each fruit you eat each day.

V: cross off a V for each vegetable you eat each day.

P.A.: write the number of minutes you participated in physical activity each day.

RDA: write a Y or N if you kept within your RDA.

There should be enough for each section, which includes three months each.

Journal Entries

Weekly Caloric Intake ______-______

Sunday 8 8 8 8 8 8 8 8

______ F F F F F V V V V V

date

P. A: ________ R.D.A.: ________

Monday 8 8 8 8 8 8 8 8

______ F F F F F V V V V V

date

P. A: ________ R.D.A.: ________

Tuesday 8 8 8 8 8 8 8 8

______ F F F F F V V V V V

date

P. A: ________ R.D.A.: ________

Wednesday 8 8 8 8 8 8 8 8

______ F F F F F V V V V V

date

P. A: ________ R.D.A.: ________

Thursday 8 8 8 8 8 8 8 8

_____ F F F F F V V V V V

date

P. A: ________ R.D.A.: ________

Friday 8 8 8 8 8 8 8 8

_____ F F F F F V V V V V

date

P. A: ________ R.D.A.: ________

Saturday 8 8 8 8 8 8 8 8

_____ F F F F F V V V V V

date

P. A: ________ R.D.A.: ________

Notes ________________________

____

____

____

____

Weekly Caloric Intake ______-______

Sunday	8 8 8 8 8 8 8 8
______	F F F F F V V V V V
date	
P. A: __________	R.D.A.: __________
Monday	8 8 8 8 8 8 8 8
______	F F F F F V V V V V
date	
P. A: __________	R.D.A.: __________
Tuesday	8 8 8 8 8 8 8 8
______	F F F F F V V V V V
date	
P. A: __________	R.D.A.: __________
Wednesday	8 8 8 8 8 8 8 8
______	F F F F F V V V V V
date	
P. A: __________	R.D.A.: __________

Thursday 8 8 8 8 8 8 8 8

______ F F F F F V V V V V

date

P. A: ________ R.D.A.: ________

Friday 8 8 8 8 8 8 8 8

______ F F F F F V V V V V

date

P. A: ________ R.D.A.: ________

Saturday 8 8 8 8 8 8 8 8

______ F F F F F V V V V V

date

P. A: ________ R.D.A.: ________

Notes ______________________________

____

____

____

____

Weekly Caloric Intake ______-______

Sunday 8 8 8 8 8 8 8 8 ______ F F F F F V V V V V date P. A: ________ R.D.A.: ________
Monday 8 8 8 8 8 8 8 8 ______ F F F F F V V V V V date P. A: ________ R.D.A.: ________
Tuesday 8 8 8 8 8 8 8 8 ______ F F F F F V V V V V date P. A: ________ R.D.A.: ________
Wednesday 8 8 8 8 8 8 8 8 ______ F F F F F V V V V V date P. A: ________ R.D.A.: ________

Thursday 8 8 8 8 8 8 8 8 _____ F F F F F V V V V V date P. A: ________ R.D.A.: ________
Friday 8 8 8 8 8 8 8 8 _____ F F F F F V V V V V date P. A: ________ R.D.A.: ________
Saturday 8 8 8 8 8 8 8 8 _____ F F F F F V V V V V date P. A: ________ R.D.A.: ________
Notes ________________________ ________________________ ________________________ ________________________ ________________________

Weekly Caloric Intake ______-______

Sunday 8 8 8 8 8 8 8 8 ______ F F F F F V V V V V date P. A: ________ R.D.A.: ________
Monday 8 8 8 8 8 8 8 8 ______ F F F F F V V V V V date P. A: ________ R.D.A.: ________
Tuesday 8 8 8 8 8 8 8 8 ______ F F F F F V V V V V date P. A: ________ R.D.A.: ________
Wednesday 8 8 8 8 8 8 8 8 ______ F F F F F V V V V V date P. A: ________ R.D.A.: ________

Thursday 8 8 8 8 8 8 8 8

______ F F F F F V V V V V

date

P. A: ________ R.D.A.: ________

Friday 8 8 8 8 8 8 8 8

______ F F F F F V V V V V

date

P. A: ________ R.D.A.: ________

Saturday 8 8 8 8 8 8 8 8

______ F F F F F V V V V V

date

P. A: ________ R.D.A.: ________

Notes ________________________

Monthly Physical Activity

Log for: ______________________________

Next to each day of the week, write the total number of minutes you engaged in physical activity that day.

1	2	3	4

5	6	7	8

9	10	11	12

13	14	15	16

17	18	19	20

21	22	23	24

25	26	27	28

29	30	31	

Monthly Total = ______________

Weekly Caloric Intake ______-______

Sunday 8 8 8 8 8 8 8 8 ______ F F F F F V V V V V date P. A: ________ R.D.A.: ________
Monday 8 8 8 8 8 8 8 8 ______ F F F F F V V V V V date P. A: ________ R.D.A.: ________
Tuesday 8 8 8 8 8 8 8 8 ______ F F F F F V V V V V date P. A: ________ R.D.A.: ________
Wednesday 8 8 8 8 8 8 8 8 ______ F F F F F V V V V V date P. A: ________ R.D.A.: ________

Thursday 8 8 8 8 8 8 8 8

______ F F F F F V V V V V

date

P. A: ________ R.D.A.: ________

Friday 8 8 8 8 8 8 8 8

______ F F F F F V V V V V

date

P. A: ________ R.D.A.: ________

Saturday 8 8 8 8 8 8 8 8

______ F F F F F V V V V V

date

P. A: ________ R.D.A.: ________

Notes ________________________

Weekly Caloric Intake _____-_____

Sunday 8 8 8 8 8 8 8 8 _____ F F F F F V V V V V date P. A: ________ R.D.A.: ________
Monday 8 8 8 8 8 8 8 8 _____ F F F F F V V V V V date P. A: ________ R.D.A.: ________
Tuesday 8 8 8 8 8 8 8 8 _____ F F F F F V V V V V date P. A: ________ R.D.A.: ________
Wednesday 8 8 8 8 8 8 8 8 _____ F F F F F V V V V V date P. A: ________ R.D.A.: ________

Thursday	8 8 8 8 8 8 8 8
______ date	F F F F F V V V V V
P. A: ________	R.D.A.: ________
Friday	8 8 8 8 8 8 8 8
______ date	F F F F F V V V V V
P. A: ________	R.D.A.: ________
Saturday	8 8 8 8 8 8 8 8
______ date	F F F F F V V V V V
P. A: ________	R.D.A.: ________

Notes ________________________

____

____

____

____

Weekly Caloric Intake ______-______

Sunday 8 8 8 8 8 8 8 8 ______ F F F F F V V V V V date P. A: ________ R.D.A.: ________
Monday 8 8 8 8 8 8 8 8 ______ F F F F F V V V V V date P. A: ________ R.D.A.: ________
Tuesday 8 8 8 8 8 8 8 8 ______ F F F F F V V V V V date P. A: ________ R.D.A.: ________
Wednesday 8 8 8 8 8 8 8 8 ______ F F F F F V V V V V date P. A: ________ R.D.A.: ________

Thursday 8 8 8 8 8 8 8 8

______ F F F F F V V V V V

date

P. A: ________ R.D.A.: ________

Friday 8 8 8 8 8 8 8 8

______ F F F F F V V V V V

date

P. A: ________ R.D.A.: ________

Saturday 8 8 8 8 8 8 8 8

______ F F F F F V V V V V

date

P. A: ________ R.D.A.: ________

Notes ________________________

Weekly Caloric Intake ______-______

Sunday 8 8 8 8 8 8 8 8 ______ F F F F F V V V V V date P. A: ________ R.D.A.: ________
Monday 8 8 8 8 8 8 8 8 ______ F F F F F V V V V V date P. A: ________ R.D.A.: ________
Tuesday 8 8 8 8 8 8 8 8 ______ F F F F F V V V V V date P. A: ________ R.D.A.: ________
Wednesday 8 8 8 8 8 8 8 8 ______ F F F F F V V V V V date P. A: ________ R.D.A.: ________

Thursday 8 8 8 8 8 8 8 8

______ F F F F F V V V V V

date

P. A: ________ R.D.A.: ________

Friday 8 8 8 8 8 8 8 8

______ F F F F F V V V V V

date

P. A: ________ R.D.A.: ________

Saturday 8 8 8 8 8 8 8 8

______ F F F F F V V V V V

date

P. A: ________ R.D.A.: ________

Notes ________________________

____

____

____

____

Monthly Physical Activity

Log for: ___________________________

Next to each day of the week, write the total number of minutes you engaged in physical activity that day.

1	2	3	4

5	6	7	8

9	10	11	12

13	14	15	16

17	18	19	20

21	22	23	24

25	26	27	28

29	30	31	

Monthly Total = ______________

Weekly Caloric Intake ______-______

Sunday 8 8 8 8 8 8 8 8 ______ F F F F F V V V V V date P. A: ________ R.D.A.: ________
Monday 8 8 8 8 8 8 8 8 ______ F F F F F V V V V V date P. A: ________ R.D.A.: ________
Tuesday 8 8 8 8 8 8 8 8 ______ F F F F F V V V V V date P. A: ________ R.D.A.: ________
Wednesday 8 8 8 8 8 8 8 8 ______ F F F F F V V V V V date P. A: ________ R.D.A.: ________

Thursday 8 8 8 8 8 8 8 8

______ F F F F F V V V V V

date

P. A: ________ R.D.A.: ________

Friday 8 8 8 8 8 8 8 8

______ F F F F F V V V V V

date

P. A: ________ R.D.A.: ________

Saturday 8 8 8 8 8 8 8 8

______ F F F F F V V V V V

date

P. A: ________ R.D.A.: ________

Notes ________________________

Weekly Caloric Intake ______-______

Sunday 8 8 8 8 8 8 8 8 ______ F F F F F V V V V V date P. A: ________ R.D.A.: ________
Monday 8 8 8 8 8 8 8 8 ______ F F F F F V V V V V date P. A: ________ R.D.A.: ________
Tuesday 8 8 8 8 8 8 8 8 ______ F F F F F V V V V V date P. A: ________ R.D.A.: ________
Wednesday 8 8 8 8 8 8 8 8 ______ F F F F F V V V V V date P. A: ________ R.D.A.: ________

Thursday 8 8 8 8 8 8 8 8

______ F F F F F V V V V V

date

P. A: ________ R.D.A.: ________

Friday 8 8 8 8 8 8 8 8

______ F F F F F V V V V V

date

P. A: ________ R.D.A.: ________

Saturday 8 8 8 8 8 8 8 8

______ F F F F F V V V V V

date

P. A: ________ R.D.A.: ________

Notes ________________________

____

____

____

____

Weekly Caloric Intake ______-______

Sunday 8 8 8 8 8 8 8 8 ______ F F F F F V V V V V date P. A: ________ R.D.A.: ________
Monday 8 8 8 8 8 8 8 8 ______ F F F F F V V V V V date P. A: ________ R.D.A.: ________
Tuesday 8 8 8 8 8 8 8 8 ______ F F F F F V V V V V date P. A: ________ R.D.A.: ________
Wednesday 8 8 8 8 8 8 8 8 ______ F F F F F V V V V V date P. A: ________ R.D.A.: ________

Thursday 8 8 8 8 8 8 8 8

______ F F F F F V V V V V

date

P. A: ________ R.D.A.: ________

Friday 8 8 8 8 8 8 8 8

______ F F F F F V V V V V

date

P. A: ________ R.D.A.: ________

Saturday 8 8 8 8 8 8 8 8

______ F F F F F V V V V V

date

P. A: ________ R.D.A.: ________

Notes ________________________

____

____

____

____

Weekly Caloric Intake ______-______

Sunday 8 8 8 8 8 8 8 8

______ F F F F F V V V V V

date

P. A: ________ R.D.A.: ________

Monday 8 8 8 8 8 8 8 8

______ F F F F F V V V V V

date

P. A: ________ R.D.A.: ________

Tuesday 8 8 8 8 8 8 8 8

______ F F F F F V V V V V

date

P. A: ________ R.D.A.: ________

Wednesday 8 8 8 8 8 8 8 8

______ F F F F F V V V V V

date

P. A: ________ R.D.A.: ________

Thursday 8 8 8 8 8 8 8 8

______ F F F F F V V V V V

date

P. A: ________ R.D.A.: ________

Friday 8 8 8 8 8 8 8 8

______ F F F F F V V V V V

date

P. A: ________ R.D.A.: ________

Saturday 8 8 8 8 8 8 8 8

______ F F F F F V V V V V

date

P. A: ________ R.D.A.: ________

Notes ________________________

Monthly Physical Activity

Log for: ___________________________

Next to each day of the week, write the total number of minutes you engaged in physical activity that day.

1	2	3	4

5	6	7	8

9	10	11	12

13	14	15	16

17	18	19	20

21	22	23	24

25	26	27	28

29	30	31	

Monthly Total = ________________

Weekly Caloric Intake ______-______

Sunday 8 8 8 8 8 8 8 8 ______ F F F F F V V V V V date P. A: ________ R.D.A.: ________
Monday 8 8 8 8 8 8 8 8 ______ F F F F F V V V V V date P. A: ________ R.D.A.: ________
Tuesday 8 8 8 8 8 8 8 8 ______ F F F F F V V V V V date P. A: ________ R.D.A.: ________
Wednesday 8 8 8 8 8 8 8 8 ______ F F F F F V V V V V date P. A: ________ R.D.A.: ________

Thursday 88888888

______ FFFFF VVVVV

date

P. A: ________ R.D.A.: ________

Friday 88888888

______ FFFFF VVVVV

date

P. A: ________ R.D.A.: ________

Saturday 88888888

______ FFFFF VVVVV

date

P. A: ________ R.D.A.: ________

Notes ________________________

____

____

____

____

Section 2

Dates

_______ to _______

Goals on Your Healthy for Life Journey

Goals

Check the box when a goal is achieved, and write the date it was achieved on the line next to the box. Write a goal next to the number, keeping in mind the ABCs.

Date
Achieved Goal

☐______ 1. ____

☐______ 2. ____

☐______ 3. ____

☐______ 4. ____

Measurement of *You* on Your Healthy for Life Journey

Date: ______________________

Location	Measurement
Neck	
Chest	
Bicep	
Waist	
Hips	
Thighs	
Weight	
BMI	

Picture of *You* on Your Healthy for Life Journey

Date: ____________________

Body Mass Index (BMI)

What is a body mass index or BMI? A BMI is an inexpensive, easy-to-perform, and reliable indicator of how much body fat a person is carrying on his or her body. To calculate your BMI, you will need the following information:

- Date of birth
- Date of measurement (the date height and weight were taken)
- Sex
- Height to nearest eighth inch
- Weight to nearest quarter pound

A BMI includes four weight-status categories as follows:

Body Mass Index Weight Status Category – Percentile Range

Weight Status Category	Percentile Range
Underweight	Less than the 5th percentile
Healthy weight	5th percentile to less than the 85th percentile
Overweight	85th to less than the 95th percentile
Obese	Equal to or greater than the 95th percentile

Source: CDC

To find your specific BMI, according to your height, weight, age, and gender, you can go to the following website at the Centers for Disease Control (CDC) and Prevention: *http://apps.nccd.cdc.gov/dnpabmi/*

Recommended Daily Allowance

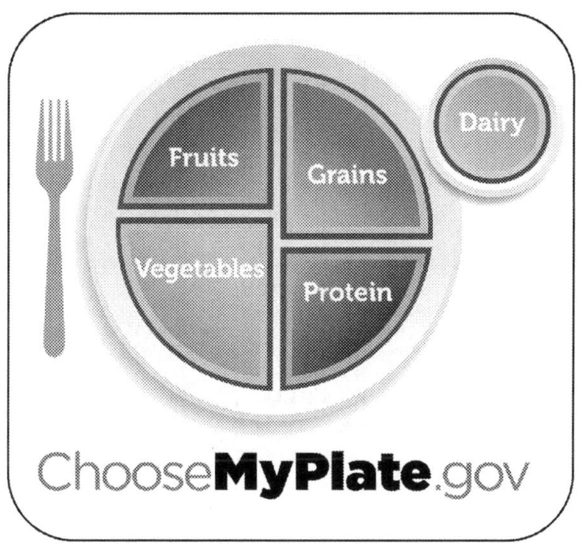

Go to the following website: www.choosemyplate.gov to find out what your recommend daily allowance (RDA), or caloric intake, should include and write it down.

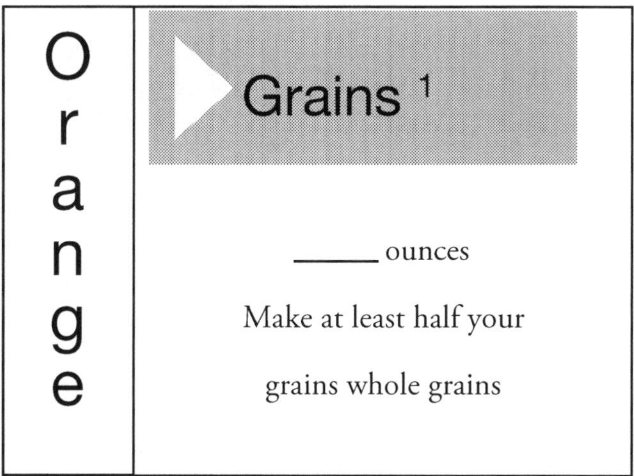

Green	**Vegetables** [2] _____ cups Try to include: dark green, red, & orange; beans & peas, starchy, & other veggies
Red	**Fruits** _____ cups Select fresh, frozen, canned, & dried fruit more often than juie
Blue	**Dairy** _____ cups Include fat-free and low-fat dairy foods every day

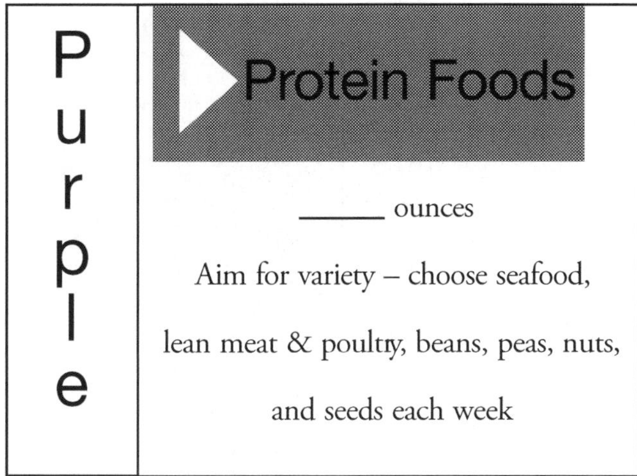

In a few months, go back to see if this has changed. As you begin to include more physical activity and your weight decreases to a healthier weight, these numbers may change.

Weekly Calorie Intake

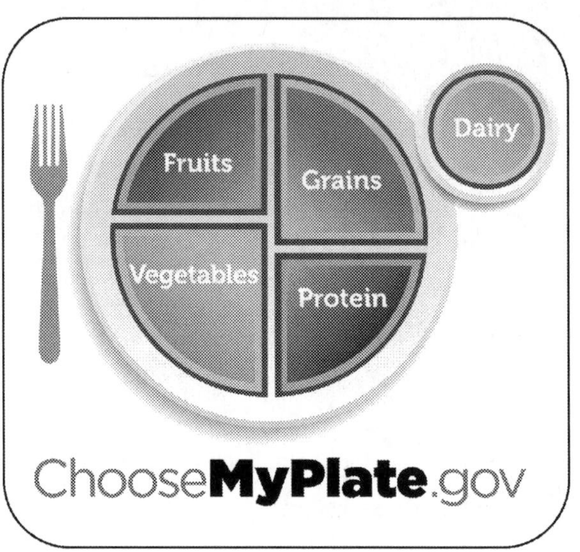

Weekly include:

Dark Green Vegetables: _____ cups

Orange Vegetables: _____ cups

Dry Beans & Peas: _____ cups

Starchy Vegetables: _____ cups

Other Vegetables: _____ cups

New Foods I will try this quarter

Grains: ______________________ ______________________ ______________________
Vegetables: ______________________ ______________________ ______________________
Fruits: ______________________ ______________________ ______________________
Dairy: ______________________ ______________________ ______________________
Protein: ______________________ ______________________ ______________________

How to use your weekly caloric intake log:

Write the date under the day of the week.

8: cross off an 8 for each eight ounces of water you drink each day.

F: cross off an F for each fruit you eat each day.

V: cross off a V for each vegetable you eat each day.

P.A.: write the number of minutes you participated in physical activity each day.

RDA: write a Y or N if you kept within your RDA.

There should be enough for each section, which includes three months each.

Journal Entries

Weekly Caloric Intake _____-_____

Sunday 8 8 8 8 8 8 8 8

_____ F F F F F V V V V V

date

P. A: ________ R.D.A.: ________

Monday 8 8 8 8 8 8 8 8

_____ F F F F F V V V V V

date

P. A: ________ R.D.A.: ________

Tuesday 8 8 8 8 8 8 8 8

_____ F F F F F V V V V V

date

P. A: ________ R.D.A.: ________

Wednesday 8 8 8 8 8 8 8 8

_____ F F F F F V V V V V

date

P. A: ________ R.D.A.: ________

Thursday	8 8 8 8 8 8 8 8
______ date	F F F F F V V V V V
P. A: ________	R.D.A.: ________
Friday	8 8 8 8 8 8 8 8
______ date	F F F F F V V V V V
P. A: ________	R.D.A.: ________
Saturday	8 8 8 8 8 8 8 8
______ date	F F F F F V V V V V
P. A: ________	R.D.A.: ________

Notes ________________________

____

____

____

____

Weekly Caloric Intake ______-______

Sunday 8 8 8 8 8 8 8 8 ______ F F F F F V V V V V date P. A: ________ R.D.A.: ________
Monday 8 8 8 8 8 8 8 8 ______ F F F F F V V V V V date P. A: ________ R.D.A.: ________
Tuesday 8 8 8 8 8 8 8 8 ______ F F F F F V V V V V date P. A: ________ R.D.A.: ________
Wednesday 8 8 8 8 8 8 8 8 ______ F F F F F V V V V V date P. A: ________ R.D.A.: ________

Thursday 8 8 8 8 8 8 8 8

_____ F F F F F V V V V V

date

P. A: ________ R.D.A.: ________

Friday 8 8 8 8 8 8 8 8

_____ F F F F F V V V V V

date

P. A: ________ R.D.A.: ________

Saturday 8 8 8 8 8 8 8 8

_____ F F F F F V V V V V

date

P. A: ________ R.D.A.: ________

Notes ______________________

____

____

____

____

Weekly Caloric Intake ______-______

Sunday	8 8 8 8 8 8 8 8
______ date	F F F F F V V V V V
P. A: ________	R.D.A.: ________
Monday	8 8 8 8 8 8 8 8
______ date	F F F F F V V V V V
P. A: ________	R.D.A.: ________
Tuesday	8 8 8 8 8 8 8 8
______ date	F F F F F V V V V V
P. A: ________	R.D.A.: ________
Wednesday	8 8 8 8 8 8 8 8
______ date	F F F F F V V V V V
P. A: ________	R.D.A.: ________

Thursday	88888888
______	FFFFF VVVVV
date	
P. A: ________	R.D.A.: ________
Friday	**88888888**
______	FFFFF VVVVV
date	
P. A: ________	R.D.A.: ________
Saturday	**88888888**
______	FFFFF VVVVV
date	
P. A: ________	R.D.A.: ________

Notes ________________________

____

____

____

____

Weekly Caloric Intake ______-______

Sunday 8 8 8 8 8 8 8 8
______ F F F F F V V V V V
date
P. A: _________ R.D.A.: _________
Monday 8 8 8 8 8 8 8 8
______ F F F F F V V V V V
date
P. A: _________ R.D.A.: _________
Tuesday 8 8 8 8 8 8 8 8
______ F F F F F V V V V V
date
P. A: _________ R.D.A.: _________
Wednesday 8 8 8 8 8 8 8 8
______ F F F F F V V V V V
date
P. A: _________ R.D.A.: _________

Thursday 8 8 8 8 8 8 8 8

_____ F F F F F V V V V V

date

P. A: ________ R.D.A.: ________

Friday 8 8 8 8 8 8 8 8

_____ F F F F F V V V V V

date

P. A: ________ R.D.A.: ________

Saturday 8 8 8 8 8 8 8 8

_____ F F F F F V V V V V

date

P. A: ________ R.D.A.: ________

Notes ________________________

____

____

____

____

Monthly Physical Activity

Log for: ______________________________

Next to each day of the week, write the total number of minutes you engaged in physical activity that day.

1	2	3	4

5	6	7	8

9	10	11	12

13	14	15	16

17	18	19	20

21	22	23	24

25	26	27	28

29	30	31	

Monthly Total = ______________

Weekly Caloric Intake _____-_____

Sunday 8 8 8 8 8 8 8 8 _____ F F F F F V V V V V date P. A: ________ R.D.A.: ________
Monday 8 8 8 8 8 8 8 8 _____ F F F F F V V V V V date P. A: ________ R.D.A.: ________
Tuesday 8 8 8 8 8 8 8 8 _____ F F F F F V V V V V date P. A: ________ R.D.A.: ________
Wednesday 8 8 8 8 8 8 8 8 _____ F F F F F V V V V V date P. A: ________ R.D.A.: ________

Thursday 8 8 8 8 8 8 8 8 ______ F F F F F V V V V V date P. A: ________ R.D.A.: ________
Friday 8 8 8 8 8 8 8 8 ______ F F F F F V V V V V date P. A: ________ R.D.A.: ________
Saturday 8 8 8 8 8 8 8 8 ______ F F F F F V V V V V date P. A: ________ R.D.A.: ________
Notes ________________________ ______________________________ ______________________________ ______________________________ ______________________________

Weekly Caloric Intake ______-______

Sunday 8 8 8 8 8 8 8 8 ______ F F F F F V V V V V date P. A: ________ R.D.A.: ________
Monday 8 8 8 8 8 8 8 8 ______ F F F F F V V V V V date P. A: ________ R.D.A.: ________
Tuesday 8 8 8 8 8 8 8 8 ______ F F F F F V V V V V date P. A: ________ R.D.A.: ________
Wednesday 8 8 8 8 8 8 8 8 ______ F F F F F V V V V V date P. A: ________ R.D.A.: ________

Thursday 8 8 8 8 8 8 8 8

______ F F F F F V V V V V

date

P. A: ________ R.D.A.: ________

Friday 8 8 8 8 8 8 8 8

______ F F F F F V V V V V

date

P. A: ________ R.D.A.: ________

Saturday 8 8 8 8 8 8 8 8

______ F F F F F V V V V V

date

P. A: ________ R.D.A.: ________

Notes ________________________

____

____

____

____

Weekly Caloric Intake _____-_____

Sunday 8 8 8 8 8 8 8 8 _____ F F F F F V V V V V date P. A: ________ R.D.A.: ________
Monday 8 8 8 8 8 8 8 8 _____ F F F F F V V V V V date P. A: ________ R.D.A.: ________
Tuesday 8 8 8 8 8 8 8 8 _____ F F F F F V V V V V date P. A: ________ R.D.A.: ________
Wednesday 8 8 8 8 8 8 8 8 _____ F F F F F V V V V V date P. A: ________ R.D.A.: ________

Thursday 8 8 8 8 8 8 8 8

______ F F F F F V V V V V

date

P. A: ________ R.D.A.: ________

Friday 8 8 8 8 8 8 8 8

______ F F F F F V V V V V

date

P. A: ________ R.D.A.: ________

Saturday 8 8 8 8 8 8 8 8

______ F F F F F V V V V V

date

P. A: ________ R.D.A.: ________

Notes ________________________

____

____

____

____

Weekly Caloric Intake ______-______

Sunday 8 8 8 8 8 8 8 8 ______ F F F F F V V V V V date P. A: ________ R.D.A.: ________
Monday 8 8 8 8 8 8 8 8 ______ F F F F F V V V V V date P. A: ________ R.D.A.: ________
Tuesday 8 8 8 8 8 8 8 8 ______ F F F F F V V V V V date P. A: ________ R.D.A.: ________
Wednesday 8 8 8 8 8 8 8 8 ______ F F F F F V V V V V date P. A: ________ R.D.A.: ________

Thursday 8 8 8 8 8 8 8 8

_____ F F F F F V V V V V

date

P. A: ________ R.D.A.: ________

Friday 8 8 8 8 8 8 8 8

_____ F F F F F V V V V V

date

P. A: ________ R.D.A.: ________

Saturday 8 8 8 8 8 8 8 8

_____ F F F F F V V V V V

date

P. A: ________ R.D.A.: ________

Notes ________________________

____

____

____

____

Monthly Physical Activity

Log for: ______________________________

Next to each day of the week, write the total number of minutes you engaged in physical activity that day.

1	2	3	4

5	6	7	8

9	10	11	12

13	14	15	16

17	18	19	20

21	22	23	24

25	26	27	28

29	30	31	

Monthly Total = ____________

Weekly Caloric Intake ______-______

Sunday 8 8 8 8 8 8 8 8 ______ F F F F F V V V V V date P. A: ________ R.D.A.: ________
Monday 8 8 8 8 8 8 8 8 ______ F F F F F V V V V V date P. A: ________ R.D.A.: ________
Tuesday 8 8 8 8 8 8 8 8 ______ F F F F F V V V V V date P. A: ________ R.D.A.: ________
Wednesday 8 8 8 8 8 8 8 8 ______ F F F F F V V V V V date P. A: ________ R.D.A.: ________

Thursday 88888888

______ FFFFF VVVVV

date

P. A: ________ R.D.A.: ________

Friday 88888888

______ FFFFF VVVVV

date

P. A: ________ R.D.A.: ________

Saturday 88888888

______ FFFFF VVVVV

date

P. A: ________ R.D.A.: ________

Notes ________________________

____

____

____

____

Weekly Caloric Intake _____-_____

<table>
<tr><td>Sunday 8 8 8 8 8 8 8 8
_____ F F F F F V V V V V
date
P. A: ________ R.D.A.: ________</td></tr>
<tr><td>Monday 8 8 8 8 8 8 8 8
_____ F F F F F V V V V V
date
P. A: ________ R.D.A.: ________</td></tr>
<tr><td>Tuesday 8 8 8 8 8 8 8 8
_____ F F F F F V V V V V
date
P. A: ________ R.D.A.: ________</td></tr>
<tr><td>Wednesday 8 8 8 8 8 8 8 8
_____ F F F F F V V V V V
date
P. A: ________ R.D.A.: ________</td></tr>
</table>

Thursday 88888888

______ FFFFF VVVVV

date

P. A: ________ R.D.A.: ________

Friday 88888888

______ FFFFF VVVVV

date

P. A: ________ R.D.A.: ________

Saturday 88888888

______ FFFFF VVVVV

date

P. A: ________ R.D.A.: ________

Notes ________________________

Weekly Caloric Intake _____-_____

Sunday 8 8 8 8 8 8 8 8 _____ F F F F F V V V V V date P. A: ________ R.D.A.: ________
Monday 8 8 8 8 8 8 8 8 _____ F F F F F V V V V V date P. A: ________ R.D.A.: ________
Tuesday 8 8 8 8 8 8 8 8 _____ F F F F F V V V V V date P. A: ________ R.D.A.: ________
Wednesday 8 8 8 8 8 8 8 8 _____ F F F F F V V V V V date P. A: ________ R.D.A.: ________

Thursday 8 8 8 8 8 8 8 8

______ F F F F F V V V V V

date

P. A: ________ R.D.A.: ________

Friday 8 8 8 8 8 8 8 8

______ F F F F F V V V V V

date

P. A: ________ R.D.A.: ________

Saturday 8 8 8 8 8 8 8 8

______ F F F F F V V V V V

date

P. A: ________ R.D.A.: ________

Notes ________________________

____

____

____

____

Weekly Caloric Intake _____-_____

Sunday 8 8 8 8 8 8 8 8 _____ F F F F F V V V V V date P. A: ________ R.D.A.: ________
Monday 8 8 8 8 8 8 8 8 _____ F F F F F V V V V V date P. A: ________ R.D.A.: ________
Tuesday 8 8 8 8 8 8 8 8 _____ F F F F F V V V V V date P. A: ________ R.D.A.: ________
Wednesday 8 8 8 8 8 8 8 8 _____ F F F F F V V V V V date P. A: ________ R.D.A.: ________

Thursday 8 8 8 8 8 8 8 8

______ F F F F F V V V V V

date

P. A: ________ R.D.A.: ________

Friday 8 8 8 8 8 8 8 8

______ F F F F F V V V V V

date

P. A: ________ R.D.A.: ________

Saturday 8 8 8 8 8 8 8 8

______ F F F F F V V V V V

date

P. A: ________ R.D.A.: ________

Notes ________________________

____

____

____

____

Monthly Physical Activity

Log for: ______________________________

Next to each day of the week, write the total number of minutes you engaged in physical activity that day.

1	2	3	4

5	6	7	8

9	10	11	12

13	14	15	16

17	18	19	20

21	22	23	24

25	26	27	28

29	30	31	

Monthly Total = ______________

Weekly Caloric Intake _____-_____

Sunday 8 8 8 8 8 8 8 8 _____ F F F F F V V V V V date P. A: ________ R.D.A.: ________
Monday 8 8 8 8 8 8 8 8 _____ F F F F F V V V V V date P. A: ________ R.D.A.: ________
Tuesday 8 8 8 8 8 8 8 8 _____ F F F F F V V V V V date P. A: ________ R.D.A.: ________
Wednesday 8 8 8 8 8 8 8 8 _____ F F F F F V V V V V date P. A: ________ R.D.A.: ________

Thursday	8 8 8 8 8 8 8 8	
______ date	F F F F F	V V V V V
P. A: ________	R.D.A.: ________	

Friday	8 8 8 8 8 8 8 8	
______ date	F F F F F	V V V V V
P. A: ________	R.D.A.: ________	

Saturday	8 8 8 8 8 8 8 8	
______ date	F F F F F	V V V V V
P. A: ________	R.D.A.: ________	

Notes ______________________________

____

____

____

____

Section 3

Dates

_______ to _______

Goals on Your Healthy for Life Journey

Goals

> Check the box when a goal is achieved, and write the date it was achieved on the line next to the box. Write a goal next to the number, keeping in mind the ABCs.

Date
Achieved Goal

☐______ 1. ____

☐______ 2. ____

☐______ 3. ____

☐______ 4. ____

Measurement of *You* on Your Healthy for Life Journey

Date: ____________________

Location	Measurement
Neck	
Chest	
Bicep	
Waist	
Hips	
Thighs	
Weight	
BMI	

Picture of *You* on Your Healthy for Life Journey

Date: ______________________

Physical Activity

In 2010, the Centers for Disease Control (CDC, 2010) published a state indicator report on physical activity that stated *physical activity is essential to overall health*. The report listed four benefits of physical activity, stating that physical activity can help control weight, reduce the risk of heart disease and some cancers, strengthen bones and muscles, and improve mental health. For young children, physical activity has additional benefits. Physical activity also helps improve fine and gross motor skills, coordination, balance and control, hand-eye coordination, strength, dexterity, and flexibility.

The US Department of Health and Human Services and the Centers for Disease Control (2008) recommends that children and teens get a minimum of *sixty minutes of physical activity every single day*. Physical activity is defined as bodily motion resulting in energy expenditure that is produced by skeletal muscles (Schumacher & Queen, 2007).

According to the US Department of Health and Human Services, children and adolescents should participate in the following types and amounts of physical activity:

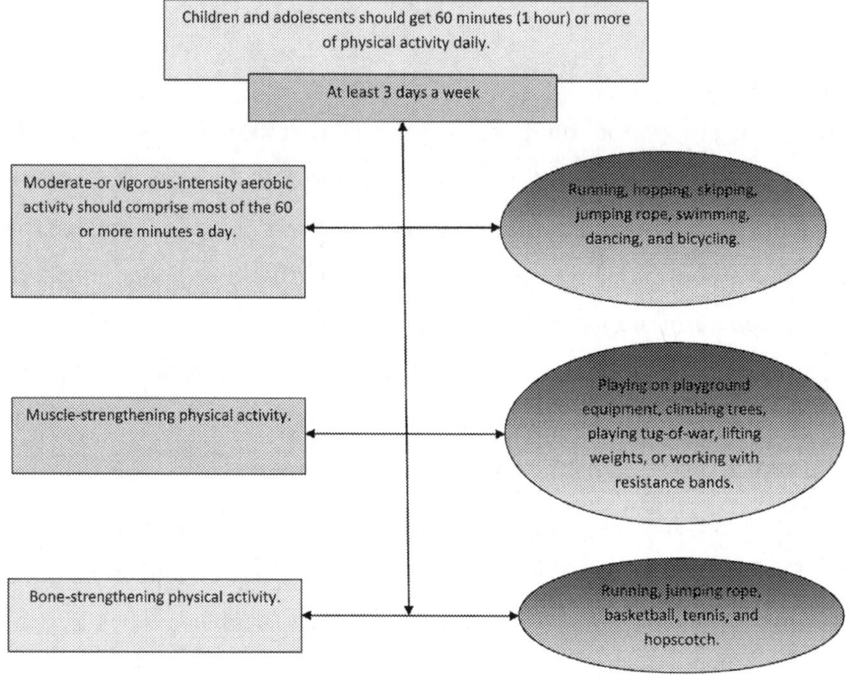

Physical Activity Guidelines for Children and Adolescents

Source: USDHHS, CDC

In addition to the sixty minutes of physical activity daily, the US Department of Health and Human Services recommends at least three days a week in the following categories: moderate- or vigorous-intensity aerobic activity, muscle-strengthening physical activity, and bone-strengthening physical activity. If you are unsure of what activities you could do for each category, here are some examples:

For moderate- or vigorous-intensity aerobic activity, you could go for a run, hop, skip, jump rope, swim, dance, or ride a bicycle.

For muscle-strengthening activities, you could play on playground equipment, climb trees, play tug-of-war, and do activities such as lifting weights or working with resistance bands.

For bone-strengthening activities, you could do some activities that were also listed in the moderate- or vigorous-intensity aerobic activity area, such as running and jumping rope, or you could also play basketball or tennis or a game of hopscotch.

Recommended Daily Allowance

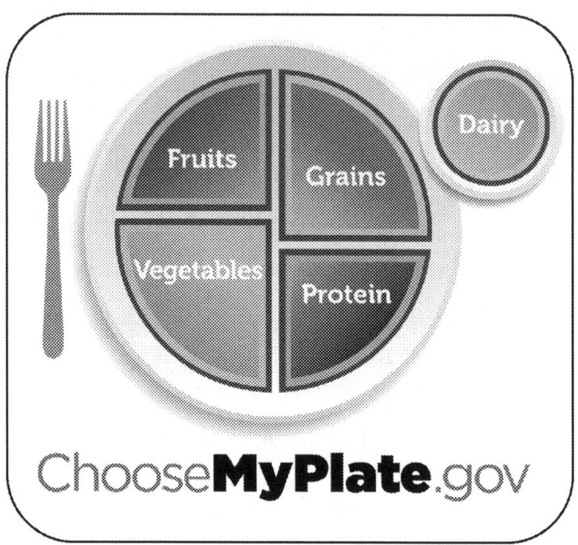

Go to the following website:
www.choosemyplate.gov to find out what your recommend daily allowance (RDA), or caloric intake, should include and write it down.

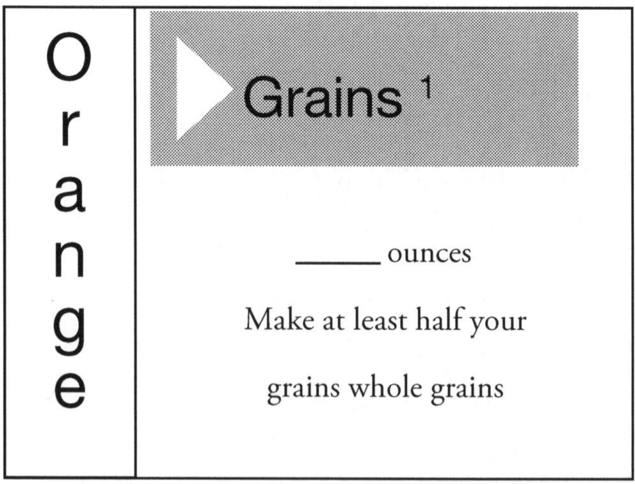

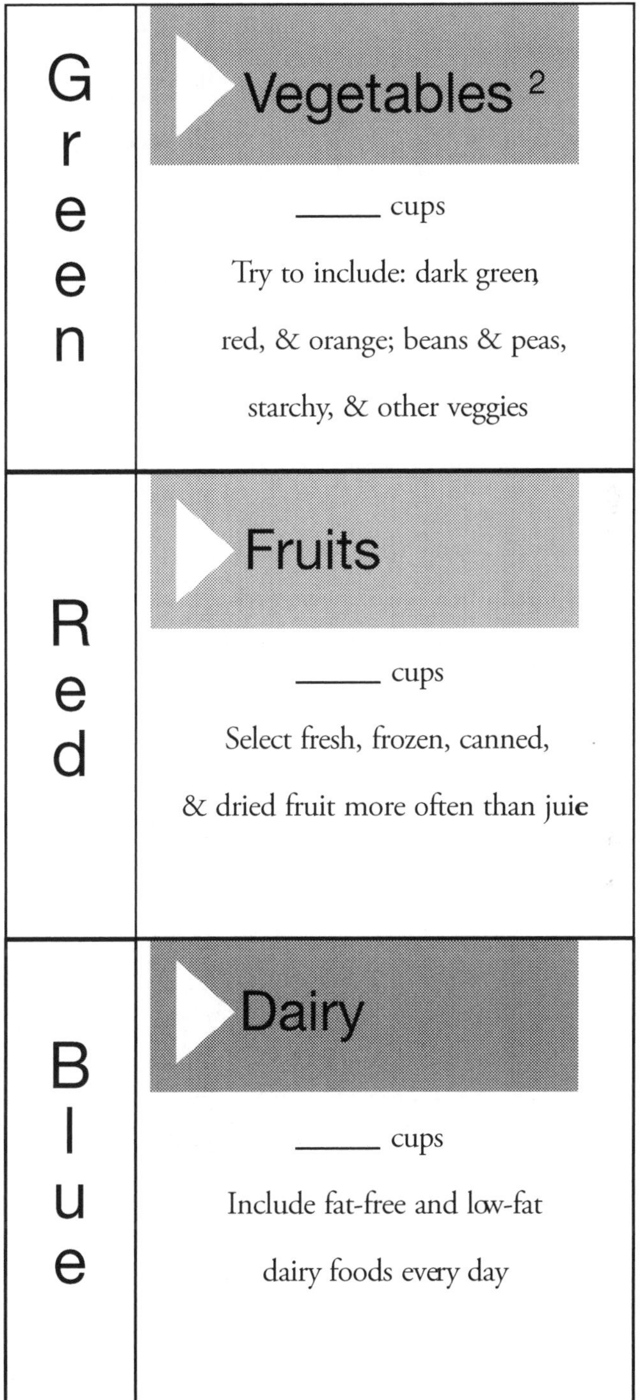

Green	**Vegetables** [2] _____ cups Try to include: dark green, red, & orange; beans & peas, starchy, & other veggies
Red	**Fruits** _____ cups Select fresh, frozen, canned, & dried fruit more often than juie
Blue	**Dairy** _____ cups Include fat-free and low-fat dairy foods every day

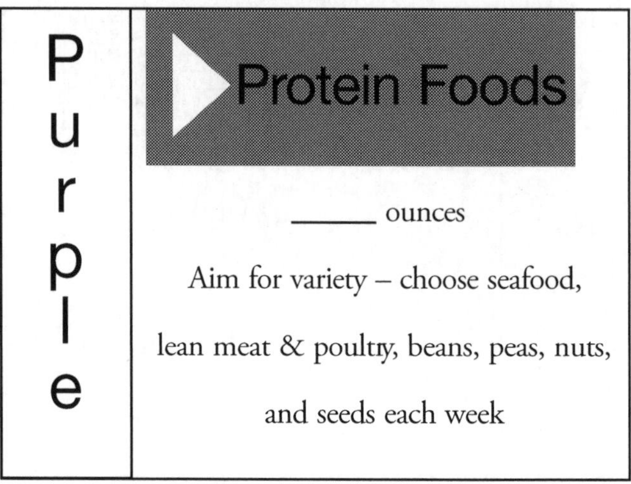

In a few months, go back to see if this has changed. As you begin to include more physical activity and your weight decreases to a healthier weight, these numbers may change.

Weekly Calorie Intake

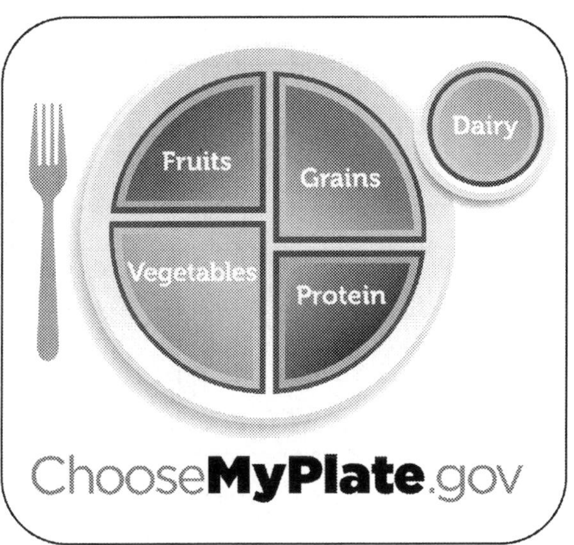

Weekly include:

Dark Green Vegetables: ______ cups

Orange Vegetables: ______ cups

Dry Beans & Peas: ______ cups

Starchy Vegetables: ______ cups

Other Vegetables: ______ cups

New Foods I will try this quarter

Grains: ______________________

____

____

Vegetables: ______________________

____

____

Fruits: ______________________

____

____

Dairy: ______________________

____

____

Protein: ______________________

____

____

How to use your weekly caloric intake log:

Write the date under the day of the week.

8: cross off an 8 for each eight ounces of water you drink each day.

F: cross off an F for each fruit you eat each day.

V: cross off a V for each vegetable you eat each day.

P.A.: write the number of minutes you participated in physical activity each day.

RDA: write a Y or N if you kept within your RDA.

There should be enough for each section, which includes three months each.

Journal Entries

Weekly Caloric Intake ______-______

Sunday 8 8 8 8 8 8 8 8 ______ F F F F F V V V V V date P. A: ________ R.D.A.: ________
Monday 8 8 8 8 8 8 8 8 ______ F F F F F V V V V V date P. A: ________ R.D.A.: ________
Tuesday 8 8 8 8 8 8 8 8 ______ F F F F F V V V V V date P. A: ________ R.D.A.: ________
Wednesday 8 8 8 8 8 8 8 8 ______ F F F F F V V V V V date P. A: ________ R.D.A.: ________

Thursday 8 8 8 8 8 8 8 8

______ F F F F F V V V V V

date

P. A: ________ R.D.A.: ________

Friday 8 8 8 8 8 8 8 8

______ F F F F F V V V V V

date

P. A: ________ R.D.A.: ________

Saturday 8 8 8 8 8 8 8 8

______ F F F F F V V V V V

date

P. A: ________ R.D.A.: ________

Notes ________________________

____

____

____

____

Weekly Caloric Intake _____-_____

Sunday	8 8 8 8 8 8 8 8
_____	F F F F F V V V V V
date	
P. A: ________	R.D.A.: ________
Monday	8 8 8 8 8 8 8 8
_____	F F F F F V V V V V
date	
P. A: ________	R.D.A.: ________
Tuesday	8 8 8 8 8 8 8 8
_____	F F F F F V V V V V
date	
P. A: ________	R.D.A.: ________
Wednesday	8 8 8 8 8 8 8 8
_____	F F F F F V V V V V
date	
P. A: ________	R.D.A.: ________

Thursday 8 8 8 8 8 8 8 8

______ F F F F F V V V V V

date

P. A: ________ R.D.A.: ________

Friday 8 8 8 8 8 8 8 8

______ F F F F F V V V V V

date

P. A: ________ R.D.A.: ________

Saturday 8 8 8 8 8 8 8 8

______ F F F F F V V V V V

date

P. A: ________ R.D.A.: ________

Notes ____________________

Weekly Caloric Intake _____-_____

Sunday 8 8 8 8 8 8 8 8 _____ F F F F F V V V V V date P. A: _______ R.D.A.: _______
Monday 8 8 8 8 8 8 8 8 _____ F F F F F V V V V V date P. A: _______ R.D.A.: _______
Tuesday 8 8 8 8 8 8 8 8 _____ F F F F F V V V V V date P. A: _______ R.D.A.: _______
Wednesday 8 8 8 8 8 8 8 8 _____ F F F F F V V V V V date P. A: _______ R.D.A.: _______

Thursday 8 8 8 8 8 8 8 8

_____ F F F F F V V V V V

date

P. A: _________ R.D.A.: _________

Friday 8 8 8 8 8 8 8 8

_____ F F F F F V V V V V

date

P. A: _________ R.D.A.: _________

Saturday 8 8 8 8 8 8 8 8

_____ F F F F F V V V V V

date

P. A: _________ R.D.A.: _________

Notes ___________________________

____

____

____

____

Weekly Caloric Intake _____-_____

Sunday 8 8 8 8 8 8 8 8 _____ F F F F F V V V V V date P. A: ________ R.D.A.: ________
Monday 8 8 8 8 8 8 8 8 _____ F F F F F V V V V V date P. A: ________ R.D.A.: ________
Tuesday 8 8 8 8 8 8 8 8 _____ F F F F F V V V V V date P. A: ________ R.D.A.: ________
Wednesday 8 8 8 8 8 8 8 8 _____ F F F F F V V V V V date P. A: ________ R.D.A.: ________

Thursday 8 8 8 8 8 8 8 8

______ F F F F F V V V V V

date

P. A: ________ R.D.A.: ________

Friday 8 8 8 8 8 8 8 8

______ F F F F F V V V V V

date

P. A: ________ R.D.A.: ________

Saturday 8 8 8 8 8 8 8 8

______ F F F F F V V V V V

date

P. A: ________ R.D.A.: ________

Notes ________________________

____

____

____

____

Monthly Physical Activity

Log for: ______________________________

Next to each day of the week, write the total number of minutes you engaged in physical activity that day.

1	2	3	4

5	6	7	8

9	10	11	12

13	14	15	16

17	18	19	20

21	22	23	24

25	26	27	28

29	30	31	

Monthly Total = ______________

Weekly Caloric Intake ______-______

Sunday 8 8 8 8 8 8 8 8 ______ F F F F F V V V V V date P. A: ________ R.D.A.: ________
Monday 8 8 8 8 8 8 8 8 ______ F F F F F V V V V V date P. A: ________ R.D.A.: ________
Tuesday 8 8 8 8 8 8 8 8 ______ F F F F F V V V V V date P. A: ________ R.D.A.: ________
Wednesday 8 8 8 8 8 8 8 8 ______ F F F F F V V V V V date P. A: ________ R.D.A.: ________

Thursday 8 8 8 8 8 8 8 8

______ F F F F F V V V V V

date

P. A: ________ R.D.A.: ________

Friday 8 8 8 8 8 8 8 8

______ F F F F F V V V V V

date

P. A: ________ R.D.A.: ________

Saturday 8 8 8 8 8 8 8 8

______ F F F F F V V V V V

date

P. A: ________ R.D.A.: ________

Notes ______________________________

____

____

____

____

Weekly Caloric Intake ______-______

Sunday 8 8 8 8 8 8 8 8 ______ F F F F F V V V V V date P. A: ________ R.D.A.: ________
Monday 8 8 8 8 8 8 8 8 ______ F F F F F V V V V V date P. A: ________ R.D.A.: ________
Tuesday 8 8 8 8 8 8 8 8 ______ F F F F F V V V V V date P. A: ________ R.D.A.: ________
Wednesday 8 8 8 8 8 8 8 8 ______ F F F F F V V V V V date P. A: ________ R.D.A.: ________

Thursday 8 8 8 8 8 8 8 8

______ F F F F F V V V V V

date

P. A: ________ R.D.A.: ________

Friday 8 8 8 8 8 8 8 8

______ F F F F F V V V V V

date

P. A: ________ R.D.A.: ________

Saturday 8 8 8 8 8 8 8 8

______ F F F F F V V V V V

date

P. A: ________ R.D.A.: ________

Notes ________________________

____

____

____

____

Weekly Caloric Intake ______-______

Sunday 8 8 8 8 8 8 8 8 ______ F F F F F V V V V V date P. A: ________ R.D.A.: ________
Monday 8 8 8 8 8 8 8 8 ______ F F F F F V V V V V date P. A: ________ R.D.A.: ________
Tuesday 8 8 8 8 8 8 8 8 ______ F F F F F V V V V V date P. A: ________ R.D.A.: ________
Wednesday 8 8 8 8 8 8 8 8 ______ F F F F F V V V V V date P. A: ________ R.D.A.: ________

Thursday 8 8 8 8 8 8 8 8

______ F F F F F V V V V V

date

P. A: ________ R.D.A.: ________

Friday 8 8 8 8 8 8 8 8

______ F F F F F V V V V V

date

P. A: ________ R.D.A.: ________

Saturday 8 8 8 8 8 8 8 8

______ F F F F F V V V V V

date

P. A: ________ R.D.A.: ________

Notes ________________________

Weekly Caloric Intake ______-______

Sunday 8 8 8 8 8 8 8 8 ______ F F F F F V V V V V date P. A: ________ R.D.A.: ________
Monday 8 8 8 8 8 8 8 8 ______ F F F F F V V V V V date P. A: ________ R.D.A.: ________
Tuesday 8 8 8 8 8 8 8 8 ______ F F F F F V V V V V date P. A: ________ R.D.A.: ________
Wednesday 8 8 8 8 8 8 8 8 ______ F F F F F V V V V V date P. A: ________ R.D.A.: ________

Thursday	8 8 8 8 8 8 8 8
______	F F F F F V V V V V
date	
P. A: ________	R.D.A.: ________
Friday	8 8 8 8 8 8 8 8
______	F F F F F V V V V V
date	
P. A: ________	R.D.A.: ________
Saturday	8 8 8 8 8 8 8 8
______	F F F F F V V V V V
date	
P. A: ________	R.D.A.: ________
Notes ________________________	
______________________________	
______________________________	
______________________________	
______________________________	

Monthly Physical Activity

Log for: ______________________________

Next to each day of the week, write the total number of minutes you engaged in physical activity that day.

1	2	3	4

5	6	7	8

9	10	11	12

13	14	15	16

17	18	19	20

21	22	23	24

25	26	27	28

29	30	31	

Monthly Total = ______________

Weekly Caloric Intake ______-______

Sunday 8 8 8 8 8 8 8 8 ______ F F F F F V V V V V date P. A: ________ R.D.A.: ________
Monday 8 8 8 8 8 8 8 8 ______ F F F F F V V V V V date P. A: ________ R.D.A.: ________
Tuesday 8 8 8 8 8 8 8 8 ______ F F F F F V V V V V date P. A: ________ R.D.A.: ________
Wednesday 8 8 8 8 8 8 8 8 ______ F F F F F V V V V V date P. A: ________ R.D.A.: ________

Thursday	8 8 8 8 8 8 8 8
______ date	F F F F F V V V V V
P. A: ________	R.D.A.: ________

Friday	8 8 8 8 8 8 8 8
______ date	F F F F F V V V V V
P. A: ________	R.D.A.: ________

Saturday	8 8 8 8 8 8 8 8
______ date	F F F F F V V V V V
P. A: ________	R.D.A.: ________

Notes ______________________

____

____

____

____

Weekly Caloric Intake _____-_____

Sunday 8 8 8 8 8 8 8 8
_____ F F F F F V V V V V
date
P. A: _______ R.D.A.: _______
Monday 8 8 8 8 8 8 8 8
_____ F F F F F V V V V V
date
P. A: _______ R.D.A.: _______
Tuesday 8 8 8 8 8 8 8 8
_____ F F F F F V V V V V
date
P. A: _______ R.D.A.: _______
Wednesday 8 8 8 8 8 8 8 8
_____ F F F F F V V V V V
date
P. A: _______ R.D.A.: _______

Thursday 8 8 8 8 8 8 8 8

______ F F F F F V V V V V

date

P. A: ________ R.D.A.: ________

Friday 8 8 8 8 8 8 8 8

______ F F F F F V V V V V

date

P. A: ________ R.D.A.: ________

Saturday 8 8 8 8 8 8 8 8

______ F F F F F V V V V V

date

P. A: ________ R.D.A.: ________

Notes ________________________

____

____

____

____

Weekly Caloric Intake ______-______

Sunday 8 8 8 8 8 8 8 8

______ F F F F F V V V V V

date

P. A: ________ R.D.A.: ________

Monday 8 8 8 8 8 8 8 8

______ F F F F F V V V V V

date

P. A: ________ R.D.A.: ________

Tuesday 8 8 8 8 8 8 8 8

______ F F F F F V V V V V

date

P. A: ________ R.D.A.: ________

Wednesday 8 8 8 8 8 8 8 8

______ F F F F F V V V V V

date

P. A: ________ R.D.A.: ________

Thursday	8 8 8 8 8 8 8 8
______ date	F F F F F V V V V V
P. A: ________	R.D.A.: ________

Friday	8 8 8 8 8 8 8 8
______ date	F F F F F V V V V V
P. A: ________	R.D.A.: ________

Saturday	8 8 8 8 8 8 8 8
______ date	F F F F F V V V V V
P. A: ________	R.D.A.: ________

Notes ________________________

____

____

____

____

Weekly Caloric Intake _____-_____

Sunday 8 8 8 8 8 8 8 8 _____ F F F F F V V V V V date P. A: _______ R.D.A.: _______
Monday 8 8 8 8 8 8 8 8 _____ F F F F F V V V V V date P. A: _______ R.D.A.: _______
Tuesday 8 8 8 8 8 8 8 8 _____ F F F F F V V V V V date P. A: _______ R.D.A.: _______
Wednesday 8 8 8 8 8 8 8 8 _____ F F F F F V V V V V date P. A: _______ R.D.A.: _______

Thursday	8 8 8 8 8 8 8 8
______ date	F F F F F V V V V V
P. A: ________	R.D.A.: ________
Friday	8 8 8 8 8 8 8 8
______ date	F F F F F V V V V V
P. A: ________	R.D.A.: ________
Saturday	8 8 8 8 8 8 8 8
______ date	F F F F F V V V V V
P. A: ________	R.D.A.: ________

Notes ______________________________

____

____

____

____

Monthly Physical Activity

Log for: ______________________________

Next to each day of the week, write the total number of minutes you engaged in physical activity that day.

1	2	3	4

5	6	7	8

9	10	11	12

13	14	15	16

17	18	19	20

21	22	23	24

25	26	27	28

29	30	31	

Monthly Total = ______________

Weekly Caloric Intake _____-_____

Sunday 8 8 8 8 8 8 8 8 _____ F F F F F V V V V V date P. A: ________ R.D.A.: ________
Monday 8 8 8 8 8 8 8 8 _____ F F F F F V V V V V date P. A: ________ R.D.A.: ________
Tuesday 8 8 8 8 8 8 8 8 _____ F F F F F V V V V V date P. A: ________ R.D.A.: ________
Wednesday 8 8 8 8 8 8 8 8 _____ F F F F F V V V V V date P. A: ________ R.D.A.: ________

Thursday	8 8 8 8 8 8 8 8
_____	F F F F F V V V V V
date	
P. A: ________	R.D.A.: ________
Friday	8 8 8 8 8 8 8 8
_____	F F F F F V V V V V
date	
P. A: ________	R.D.A.: ________
Saturday	8 8 8 8 8 8 8 8
_____	F F F F F V V V V V
date	
P. A: ________	R.D.A.: ________

Notes ______________________

____

____

____

____

Section 4

Dates

________ to ________

Goals on Your Healthy for Life Journey

Goals

> Check the box when a goal is achieved, and write the date it was achieved on the line next to the box. Write a goal next to the number, keeping in mind the ABCs.

Date
Achieved	Goal

☐______ 1. ______________________________________

☐______ 2. ______________________________________

☐______ 3. ______________________________________

☐______ 4. ______________________________________

Measurement of *You* on Your Healthy for Life Journey

Date: ______________________

Location	Measurement
Neck	
Chest	
Bicep	
Waist	
Hips	
Thighs	
Weight	
BMI	

Picture of *You* on Your Healthy for Life Journey

Date: ___________________

Eating a Rainbow Every Day

A great way to help balance your scale is to incorporate a rainbow in your daily caloric intake. This means making sure you eat fruits and vegetables every day that include all the colors of the rainbow. Fruit and vegetables provide various nutritional values according to color. Below is a list of the various colors of the rainbow—including white due to its nutritional value—with fruit and vegetable suggestions, accompanied by the nutritional values they provide.

- Purple—promotes microcirculation

  Fruits/Vegetables: grapes, plums, blackberries, raisins, eggplant, purple cabbage, onions, passion fruit, mint flowers, mulberries, lavender

- Blue-nutritional value not specifically stated

  Fruits/Vegetables: blueberries, juniper berries, blue grapes, blue potatoes, cauliflower

- Green—rejuvenates musculature and bones

  Fruits/Vegetables: spinach, kiwi, broccoli, cucumbers, celery, bell peppers, grapes, zucchini, avocado, apples, asparagus, Brussels sprouts, cactus, chives, collard greens, fennel, green beans, olives, honeydew, kale, lettuce, limes, mint, okra, Swiss chard, tarragon, tomatillo

- White—enhances immune system, lymph system, and cellular recovery

  Fruits/Vegetables: onions, bananas, cauliflower, mushrooms, coconut, jicama, shallots, turnips, garlic, horseradish, buckwheat, tofu

- Yellow—optimizes brain functions

  Fruits/Vegetables: corn, squash, pineapple, nectarines, apples, anise seed, bamboo shoots, lemons, parsnips, pears, saffron, yellow tomatoes, summer squash, star fruit.

- Orange—optimizes brain functions

  Fruits/Vegetables: carrots, peaches, oranges, cantaloupe, butternut squash, mangos, orange peppers, papayas, winter squash, tangerines, sweet potatoes, persimmons, pumpkin, apricots.

- Red—supports heart and circulatory system

  Fruits/Vegetables: watermelon, raspberries, cherries, radishes, tomatoes, apples, strawberries, cranberries, grapefruit, guava, red cabbage, red peppers, tomatoes, rhubarb

Recommended Daily Allowance

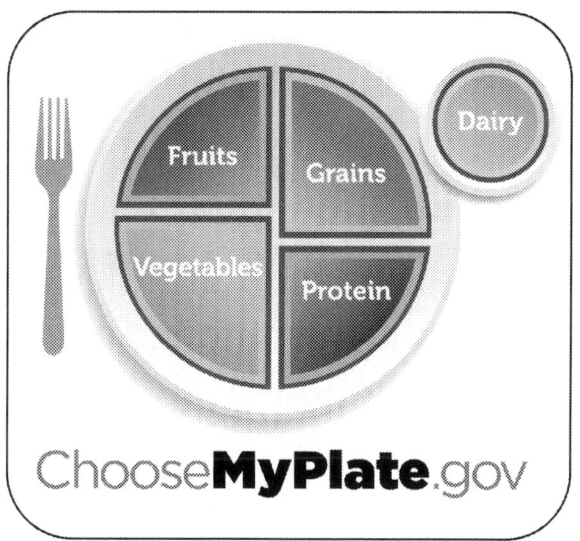

Go to the following website: www.choosemyplate.gov to find out what your recommend daily allowance (RDA), or caloric intake, should include and write it down.

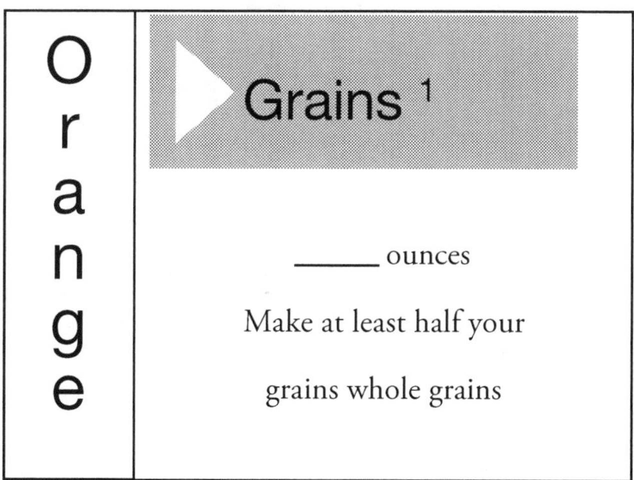

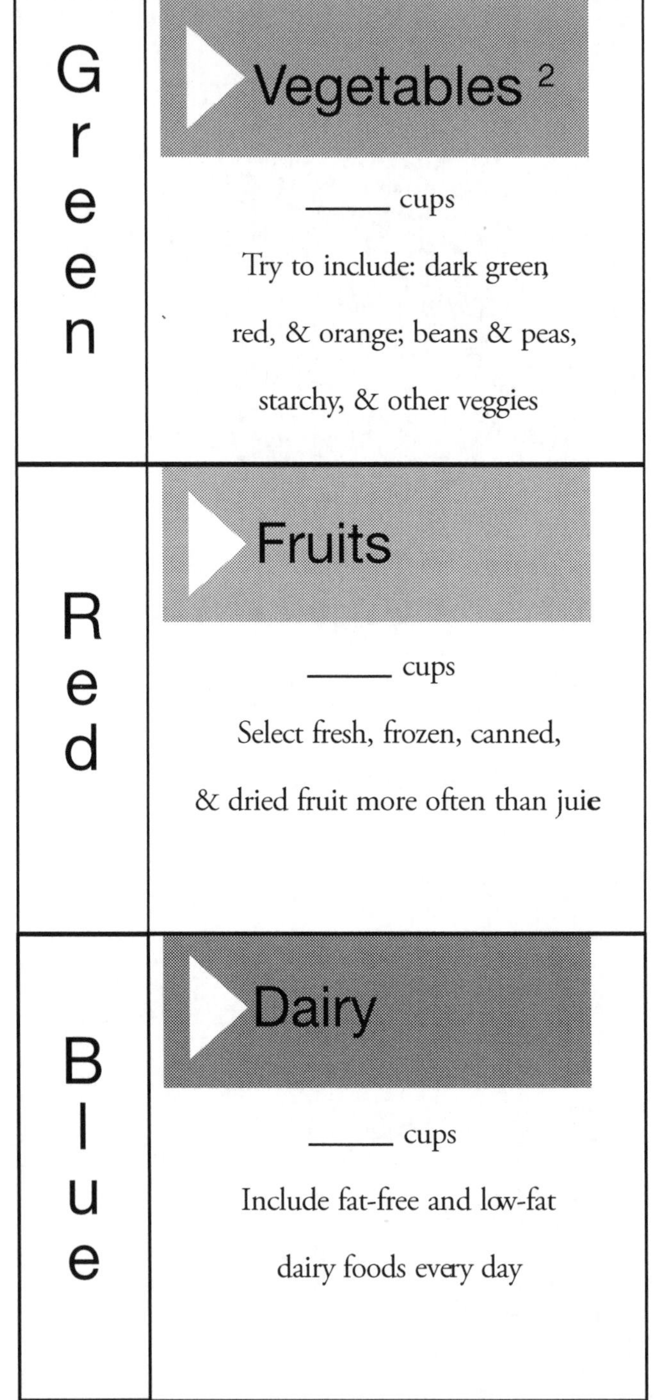
Green
Vegetables 2
_____ cups
Try to include: dark green,
red, & orange; beans & peas,
starchy, & other veggies
Red
Fruits
_____ cups
Select fresh, frozen, canned,
& dried fruit more often than juie
Blue
Dairy
_____ cups
Include fat-free and low-fat
dairy foods every day

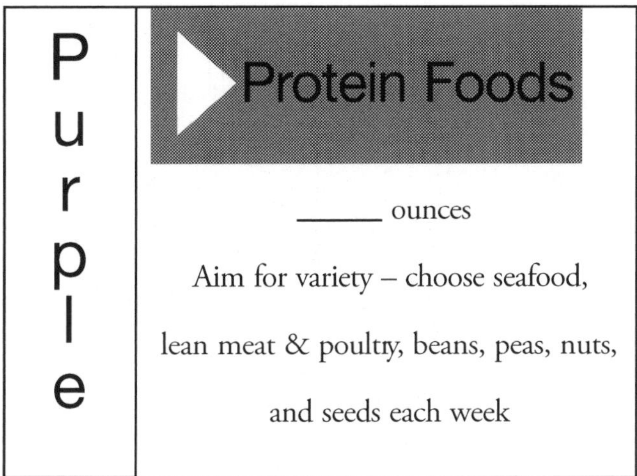

In a few months, go back to see if this has changed. As you begin to include more physical activity and your weight decreases to a healthier weight, these numbers may change.

Weekly Calorie Intake

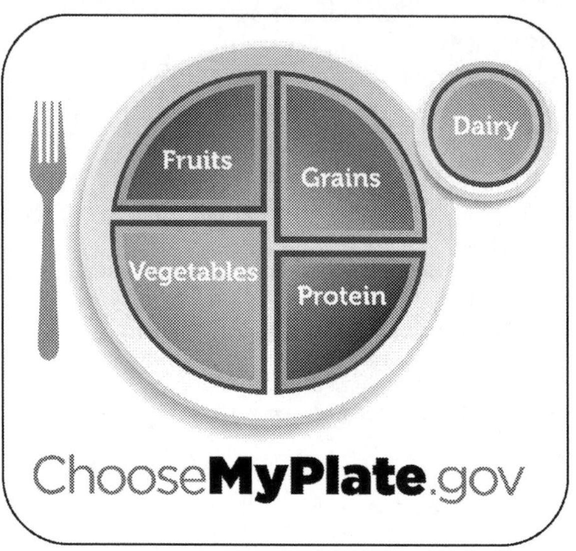

Weekly include:

Dark Green Vegetables: ______ cups

Orange Vegetables: ______ cups

Dry Beans & Peas: ______ cups

Starchy Vegetables: ______ cups

Other Vegetables: ______ cups

New Foods I will try this quarter

Grains: ______________________ ______________________ ______________________
Vegetables: ______________________ ______________________ ______________________
Fruits: ______________________ ______________________ ______________________
Dairy: ______________________ ______________________ ______________________
Protein: ______________________ ______________________ ______________________

How to use your weekly caloric intake log:

Write the date under the day of the week.

8: cross off an 8 for each eight ounces of water you drink each day.

F: cross off an F for each fruit you eat each day.

V: cross off a V for each vegetable you eat each day.

P.A.: write the number of minutes you participated in physical activity each day.

RDA: write a Y or N if you kept within your RDA.

There should be enough for each section, which includes three months each.

Journal Entries

Weekly Caloric Intake _____-_____

Sunday	8 8 8 8 8 8 8 8
_____	F F F F F V V V V V
date	
P. A: _______	R.D.A.: _______
Monday	8 8 8 8 8 8 8 8
_____	F F F F F V V V V V
date	
P. A: _______	R.D.A.: _______
Tuesday	8 8 8 8 8 8 8 8
_____	F F F F F V V V V V
date	
P. A: _______	R.D.A.: _______
Wednesday	8 8 8 8 8 8 8 8
_____	F F F F F V V V V V
date	
P. A: _______	R.D.A.: _______

Thursday 8 8 8 8 8 8 8 8

______ F F F F F V V V V V

date

P. A: ________ R.D.A.: ________

Friday 8 8 8 8 8 8 8 8

______ F F F F F V V V V V

date

P. A: ________ R.D.A.: ________

Saturday 8 8 8 8 8 8 8 8

______ F F F F F V V V V V

date

P. A: ________ R.D.A.: ________

Notes ________________________

____

____

____

____

Weekly Caloric Intake ______-______

Sunday 8 8 8 8 8 8 8 8 ______ F F F F F V V V V V date P. A: ________ R.D.A.: ________
Monday 8 8 8 8 8 8 8 8 ______ F F F F F V V V V V date P. A: ________ R.D.A.: ________
Tuesday 8 8 8 8 8 8 8 8 ______ F F F F F V V V V V date P. A: ________ R.D.A.: ________
Wednesday 8 8 8 8 8 8 8 8 ______ F F F F F V V V V V date P. A: ________ R.D.A.: ________

Thursday 8 8 8 8 8 8 8 8

______ F F F F F V V V V V

date

P. A: ________ R.D.A.: ________

Friday 8 8 8 8 8 8 8 8

______ F F F F F V V V V V

date

P. A: ________ R.D.A.: ________

Saturday 8 8 8 8 8 8 8 8

______ F F F F F V V V V V

date

P. A: ________ R.D.A.: ________

Notes ________________________

____

____

____

____

Weekly Caloric Intake ______-______

Sunday 8 8 8 8 8 8 8 8 ______ F F F F F V V V V V date P. A: ________ R.D.A.: ________
Monday 8 8 8 8 8 8 8 8 ______ F F F F F V V V V V date P. A: ________ R.D.A.: ________
Tuesday 8 8 8 8 8 8 8 8 ______ F F F F F V V V V V date P. A: ________ R.D.A.: ________
Wednesday 8 8 8 8 8 8 8 8 ______ F F F F F V V V V V date P. A: ________ R.D.A.: ________

Thursday 88888888

______ FFFFF VVVVV

date

P. A: ________ R.D.A.: ________

Friday 88888888

______ FFFFF VVVVV

date

P. A: ________ R.D.A.: ________

Saturday 88888888

______ FFFFF VVVVV

date

P. A: ________ R.D.A.: ________

Notes ________________________

____

____

____

____

Weekly Caloric Intake ______-______

Sunday 8 8 8 8 8 8 8 8 ______ F F F F F V V V V V date P. A: ________ R.D.A.: ________
Monday 8 8 8 8 8 8 8 8 ______ F F F F F V V V V V date P. A: ________ R.D.A.: ________
Tuesday 8 8 8 8 8 8 8 8 ______ F F F F F V V V V V date P. A: ________ R.D.A.: ________
Wednesday 8 8 8 8 8 8 8 8 ______ F F F F F V V V V V date P. A: ________ R.D.A.: ________

Thursday 8 8 8 8 8 8 8 8

_____ F F F F F V V V V V

date

P. A: ________ R.D.A.: ________

Friday 8 8 8 8 8 8 8 8

_____ F F F F F V V V V V

date

P. A: ________ R.D.A.: ________

Saturday 8 8 8 8 8 8 8 8

_____ F F F F F V V V V V

date

P. A: ________ R.D.A.: ________

Notes ________________________

____

____

____

____

Monthly Physical Activity

Log for: ______________________________

Next to each day of the week, write the total number of minutes you engaged in physical activity that day.

1	2	3	4

5	6	7	8

9	10	11	12

13	14	15	16

17	18	19	20

21	22	23	24

25	26	27	28

29	30	31	

Monthly Total = ______________

Weekly Caloric Intake _____-_____

Sunday 8 8 8 8 8 8 8 8 _____ F F F F F V V V V V date P. A: ________ R.D.A.: ________
Monday 8 8 8 8 8 8 8 8 _____ F F F F F V V V V V date P. A: ________ R.D.A.: ________
Tuesday 8 8 8 8 8 8 8 8 _____ F F F F F V V V V V date P. A: ________ R.D.A.: ________
Wednesday 8 8 8 8 8 8 8 8 _____ F F F F F V V V V V date P. A: ________ R.D.A.: ________

Thursday 8 8 8 8 8 8 8 8

______ F F F F F V V V V V

date

P. A: ________ R.D.A.: ________

Friday 8 8 8 8 8 8 8 8

______ F F F F F V V V V V

date

P. A: ________ R.D.A.: ________

Saturday 8 8 8 8 8 8 8 8

______ F F F F F V V V V V

date

P. A: ________ R.D.A.: ________

Notes ________________________

____

____

____

____

Weekly Caloric Intake _____-_____

Sunday 8 8 8 8 8 8 8 8 _____ F F F F F V V V V V date P. A: _______ R.D.A.: _______
Monday 8 8 8 8 8 8 8 8 _____ F F F F F V V V V V date P. A: _______ R.D.A.: _______
Tuesday 8 8 8 8 8 8 8 8 _____ F F F F F V V V V V date P. A: _______ R.D.A.: _______
Wednesday 8 8 8 8 8 8 8 8 _____ F F F F F V V V V V date P. A: _______ R.D.A.: _______

Thursday 8 8 8 8 8 8 8 8

______ F F F F F V V V V V

date

P. A: ________ R.D.A.: ________

Friday 8 8 8 8 8 8 8 8

______ F F F F F V V V V V

date

P. A: ________ R.D.A.: ________

Saturday 8 8 8 8 8 8 8 8

______ F F F F F V V V V V

date

P. A: ________ R.D.A.: ________

Notes ________________________

____

____

____

____

Weekly Caloric Intake _____-_____

Sunday 8 8 8 8 8 8 8 8 _____ F F F F F V V V V V date P. A: _______ R.D.A.: _______
Monday 8 8 8 8 8 8 8 8 _____ F F F F F V V V V V date P. A: _______ R.D.A.: _______
Tuesday 8 8 8 8 8 8 8 8 _____ F F F F F V V V V V date P. A: _______ R.D.A.: _______
Wednesday 8 8 8 8 8 8 8 8 _____ F F F F F V V V V V date P. A: _______ R.D.A.: _______

Thursday 8 8 8 8 8 8 8 8

______ F F F F F V V V V V

date

P. A: ________ R.D.A.: ________

Friday 8 8 8 8 8 8 8 8

______ F F F F F V V V V V

date

P. A: ________ R.D.A.: ________

Saturday 8 8 8 8 8 8 8 8

______ F F F F F V V V V V

date

P. A: ________ R.D.A.: ________

Notes ________________________

____

____

____

____

Weekly Caloric Intake ______-______

Sunday 8 8 8 8 8 8 8 8 ______ F F F F F V V V V V date P. A: ________ R.D.A.: ________
Monday 8 8 8 8 8 8 8 8 ______ F F F F F V V V V V date P. A: ________ R.D.A.: ________
Tuesday 8 8 8 8 8 8 8 8 ______ F F F F F V V V V V date P. A: ________ R.D.A.: ________
Wednesday 8 8 8 8 8 8 8 8 ______ F F F F F V V V V V date P. A: ________ R.D.A.: ________

Thursday 8 8 8 8 8 8 8 8

______ F F F F F V V V V V

date

P. A: ________ R.D.A.: ________

Friday 8 8 8 8 8 8 8 8

______ F F F F F V V V V V

date

P. A: ________ R.D.A.: ________

Saturday 8 8 8 8 8 8 8 8

______ F F F F F V V V V V

date

P. A: ________ R.D.A.: ________

Notes ________________________

____

____

____

____

Monthly Physical Activity

Log for: ______________________________

Next to each day of the week, write the total number of minutes you engaged in physical activity that day.

1	2	3	4

5	6	7	8

9	10	11	12

13	14	15	16

17	18	19	20

21	22	23	24

25	26	27	28

29	30	31	

Monthly Total = ____________

Weekly Caloric Intake ______-______

Sunday 8 8 8 8 8 8 8 8 ______ F F F F F V V V V V date P. A: ________ R.D.A.: ________
Monday 8 8 8 8 8 8 8 8 ______ F F F F F V V V V V date P. A: ________ R.D.A.: ________
Tuesday 8 8 8 8 8 8 8 8 ______ F F F F F V V V V V date P. A: ________ R.D.A.: ________
Wednesday 8 8 8 8 8 8 8 8 ______ F F F F F V V V V V date P. A: ________ R.D.A.: ________

Thursday 8 8 8 8 8 8 8 8

______ F F F F F V V V V V

date

P. A: ________ R.D.A.: ________

Friday 8 8 8 8 8 8 8 8

______ F F F F F V V V V V

date

P. A: ________ R.D.A.: ________

Saturday 8 8 8 8 8 8 8 8

______ F F F F F V V V V V

date

P. A: ________ R.D.A.: ________

Notes ________________________

____

____

____

____

Weekly Caloric Intake _____-_____

Sunday 8 8 8 8 8 8 8 8 _____ F F F F F V V V V V date P. A: ________ R.D.A.: ________
Monday 8 8 8 8 8 8 8 8 _____ F F F F F V V V V V date P. A: ________ R.D.A.: ________
Tuesday 8 8 8 8 8 8 8 8 _____ F F F F F V V V V V date P. A: ________ R.D.A.: ________
Wednesday 8 8 8 8 8 8 8 8 _____ F F F F F V V V V V date P. A: ________ R.D.A.: ________

Thursday	8 8 8 8 8 8 8 8
______ date	F F F F F V V V V V
P. A: ________	R.D.A.: ________
Friday	8 8 8 8 8 8 8 8
______ date	F F F F F V V V V V
P. A: ________	R.D.A.: ________
Saturday	8 8 8 8 8 8 8 8
______ date	F F F F F V V V V V
P. A: ________	R.D.A.: ________

Notes ________________________

____

____

____

____

Weekly Caloric Intake _____-_____

Sunday 8 8 8 8 8 8 8 8 _____ F F F F F V V V V V date P. A: ________ R.D.A.: ________
Monday 8 8 8 8 8 8 8 8 _____ F F F F F V V V V V date P. A: ________ R.D.A.: ________
Tuesday 8 8 8 8 8 8 8 8 _____ F F F F F V V V V V date P. A: ________ R.D.A.: ________
Wednesday 8 8 8 8 8 8 8 8 _____ F F F F F V V V V V date P. A: ________ R.D.A.: ________

Thursday 8 8 8 8 8 8 8 8

______ F F F F F V V V V V

date

P. A: ________ R.D.A.: ________

Friday 8 8 8 8 8 8 8 8

______ F F F F F V V V V V

date

P. A: ________ R.D.A.: ________

Saturday 8 8 8 8 8 8 8 8

______ F F F F F V V V V V

date

P. A: ________ R.D.A.: ________

Notes ________________________

Weekly Caloric Intake _____-_____

Sunday 8 8 8 8 8 8 8 8 _____ F F F F F V V V V V date P. A: _______ R.D.A.: _______
Monday 8 8 8 8 8 8 8 8 _____ F F F F F V V V V V date P. A: _______ R.D.A.: _______
Tuesday 8 8 8 8 8 8 8 8 _____ F F F F F V V V V V date P. A: _______ R.D.A.: _______
Wednesday 8 8 8 8 8 8 8 8 _____ F F F F F V V V V V date P. A: _______ R.D.A.: _______

Thursday 8 8 8 8 8 8 8 8

______ F F F F F V V V V V

date

P. A: ________ R.D.A.: ________

Friday 8 8 8 8 8 8 8 8

______ F F F F F V V V V V

date

P. A: ________ R.D.A.: ________

Saturday 8 8 8 8 8 8 8 8

______ F F F F F V V V V V

date

P. A: ________ R.D.A.: ________

Notes ________________________

____

____

____

____

Monthly Physical Activity

Log for: ________________________________

Next to each day of the week, write the total number of minutes you engaged in physical activity that day.

1	2	3	4

5	6	7	8

9	10	11	12

13	14	15	16

17	18	19	20

21	22	23	24

25	26	27	28

29	30	31	

Monthly Total = ______________

Weekly Caloric Intake ______-______

Sunday 8 8 8 8 8 8 8 8 ______ F F F F F V V V V V date P. A: ________ R.D.A.: ________
Monday 8 8 8 8 8 8 8 8 ______ F F F F F V V V V V date P. A: ________ R.D.A.: ________
Tuesday 8 8 8 8 8 8 8 8 ______ F F F F F V V V V V date P. A: ________ R.D.A.: ________
Wednesday 8 8 8 8 8 8 8 8 ______ F F F F F V V V V V date P. A: ________ R.D.A.: ________

Thursday 8 8 8 8 8 8 8 8

______ F F F F F V V V V V

date

P. A: ________ R.D.A.: ________

Friday 8 8 8 8 8 8 8 8

______ F F F F F V V V V V

date

P. A: ________ R.D.A.: ________

Saturday 8 8 8 8 8 8 8 8

______ F F F F F V V V V V

date

P. A: ________ R.D.A.: ________

Notes ________________________

Section 5

Dates

________ to ________

Goals on Your Healthy for Life Journey

Goals

> Check the box when a goal is achieved, and write the date it was achieved on the line next to the box. Write a goal next to the number, keeping in mind the ABCs.

Date
Achieved Goal

☐______ 1. ____

☐______ 2. ____

☐______ 3. ____

☐______ 4. ____

Measurement of *You* on Your Healthy for Life Journey

Date: ____________________

Location	Measurement
Neck	
Chest	
Bicep	
Waist	
Hips	
Thighs	
Weight	
BMI	

Picture of *You* on Your Healthy for Life Journey

Date: ____________________

Portion Size vs. Serving Size

What exactly are portion sizes and serving sizes? And what are the differences between the two? According to the US Department of Agriculture (USDA), "a serving size is a unit of measure used to describe the amount of food recommended for each food group." A *portion size,* on the other hand, is "the amount of food eaten" and can be as big as you choose (which is where you need portion control). Therefore, it is very important that you understand the difference between serving size and portion size and document it correctly.

If you go to a buffet and write down that you ate chicken, corn on the cob, broccoli, and an apple, to determine how many calories you consumed, you need to know how much of each item you ate. To determine how much you ate or how many servings you ate in your portion size, you need to get into the habit of weighing and measuring your foods; otherwise, how will you know if you ate a cup of broccoli or if you ate six ounces of meat? Do not get confused between serving size and portion size.

Before we leave the topic of portion sizes, I want to note that portion sizes have grown a great deal over the last twenty years—no pun intended. A cheeseburger at a fast-food joint twenty years ago was roughly 330 calories; today it is almost 600! An order of spaghetti and meatballs included a cup of spaghetti, about three meatballs, and came to about 500 calories, whereas today an order of spaghetti and meatballs is over 1,000 calories.

Being from Texas, I have seen Texas-size orders, and boy, those calories are high. (I think there are even calories in just smelling some of the food!) The important thing here is not only keeping track of the portion size but also keeping *control* of those portion sizes. Often one of the best things to do is order a to-go box when you order your meal; that way at least you can spread your calories over two meals. Again, being aware of this will help you on your journey to being healthy for life.

Recommended Daily Allowance

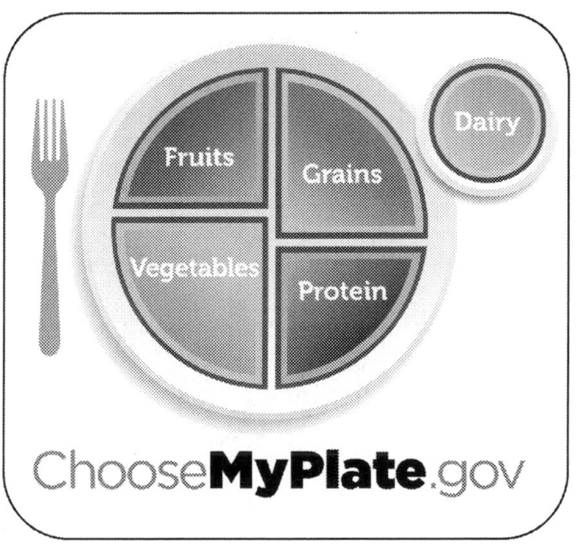

Go to the following website: www.choosemyplate.gov to find out what your recommend daily allowance (RDA), or caloric intake, should include and write it down.

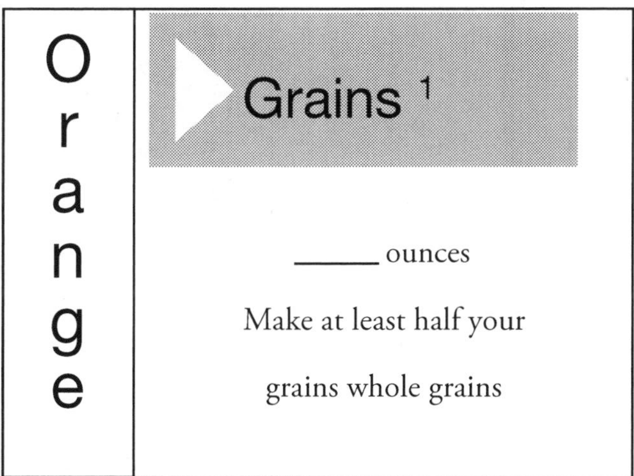

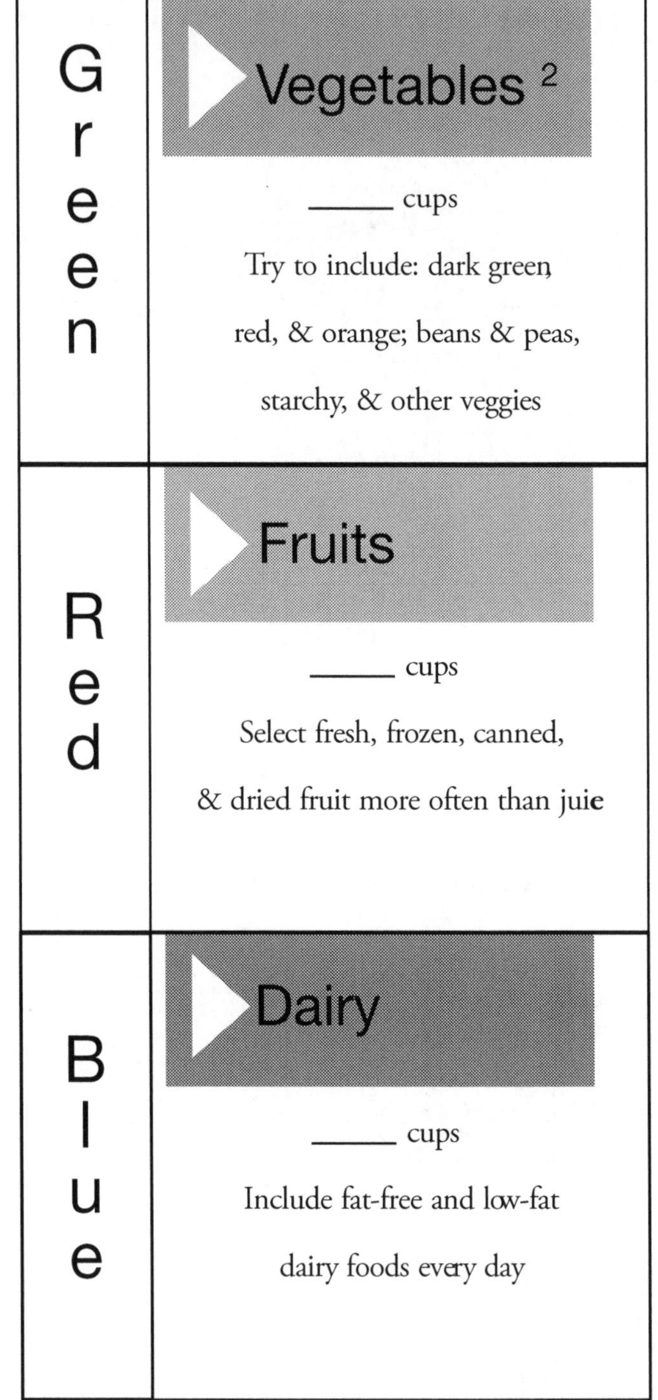

G r e e n
Vegetables [2]
_____ cups
Try to include: dark green, red, & orange; beans & peas, starchy, & other veggies
R e d
Fruits
_____ cups
Select fresh, frozen, canned, & dried fruit more often than juie
B l u e
Dairy
_____ cups
Include fat-free and low-fat dairy foods every day

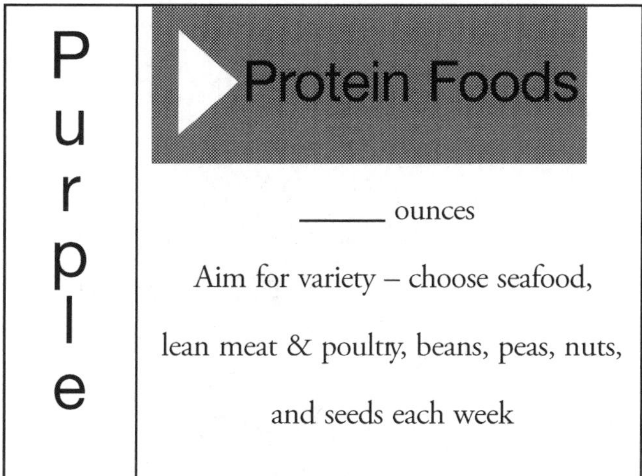

In a few months, go back to see if this has changed. As you begin to include more physical activity and your weight decreases to a healthier weight, these numbers may change.

Weekly Calorie Intake

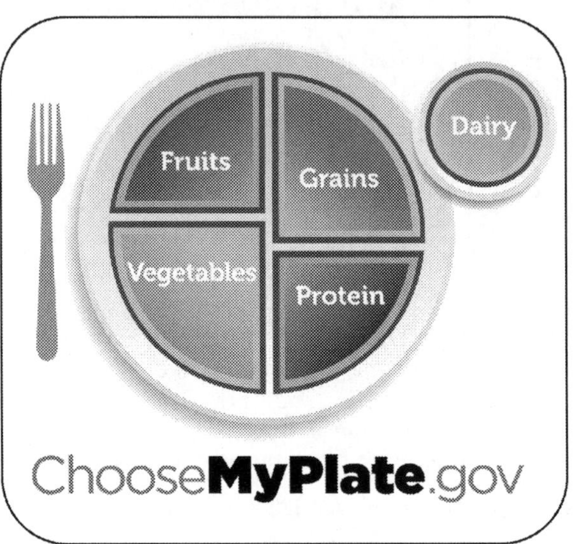

Weekly include:

Dark Green Vegetables: ______ cups

Orange Vegetables: ______ cups

Dry Beans & Peas: ______ cups

Starchy Vegetables: ______ cups

Other Vegetables: ______ cups

New Foods I will try this quarter

Grains: ____________________

____

____

Vegetables: ____________________

____

____

Fruits: ____________________

____

____

Dairy: ____________________

____

____

Protein: ____________________

____

____

How to use your weekly caloric intake log:

Write the date under the day of the week.

8: cross off an 8 for each eight ounces of water you drink each day.

F: cross off an F for each fruit you eat each day.

V: cross off a V for each vegetable you eat each day.

P.A.: write the number of minutes you participated in physical activity each day.

RDA: write a Y or N if you kept within your RDA.

There should be enough for each section, which includes three months each.

Journal Entries

Weekly Caloric Intake ______-______

Sunday 8 8 8 8 8 8 8 8 ______ F F F F F V V V V V date P. A: ________ R.D.A.: ________
Monday 8 8 8 8 8 8 8 8 ______ F F F F F V V V V V date P. A: ________ R.D.A.: ________
Tuesday 8 8 8 8 8 8 8 8 ______ F F F F F V V V V V date P. A: ________ R.D.A.: ________
Wednesday 8 8 8 8 8 8 8 8 ______ F F F F F V V V V V date P. A: ________ R.D.A.: ________

Thursday 8 8 8 8 8 8 8 8

______ F F F F F V V V V V

date

P. A: ________ R.D.A.: ________

Friday 8 8 8 8 8 8 8 8

______ F F F F F V V V V V

date

P. A: ________ R.D.A.: ________

Saturday 8 8 8 8 8 8 8 8

______ F F F F F V V V V V

date

P. A: ________ R.D.A.: ________

Notes ________________________

Weekly Caloric Intake ______-______

Sunday 8 8 8 8 8 8 8 8 ______ F F F F F V V V V V date P. A: ________ R.D.A.: ________
Monday 8 8 8 8 8 8 8 8 ______ F F F F F V V V V V date P. A: ________ R.D.A.: ________
Tuesday 8 8 8 8 8 8 8 8 ______ F F F F F V V V V V date P. A: ________ R.D.A.: ________
Wednesday 8 8 8 8 8 8 8 8 ______ F F F F F V V V V V date P. A: ________ R.D.A.: ________

Thursday 8 8 8 8 8 8 8 8

______ F F F F F V V V V V

date

P. A: ________ R.D.A.: ________

Friday 8 8 8 8 8 8 8 8

______ F F F F F V V V V V

date

P. A: ________ R.D.A.: ________

Saturday 8 8 8 8 8 8 8 8

______ F F F F F V V V V V

date

P. A: ________ R.D.A.: ________

Notes ________________________

____

____

____

____

Weekly Caloric Intake ______-______

Sunday 8 8 8 8 8 8 8 8 ______ F F F F F V V V V V date P. A: ________ R.D.A.: ________
Monday 8 8 8 8 8 8 8 8 ______ F F F F F V V V V V date P. A: ________ R.D.A.: ________
Tuesday 8 8 8 8 8 8 8 8 ______ F F F F F V V V V V date P. A: ________ R.D.A.: ________
Wednesday 8 8 8 8 8 8 8 8 ______ F F F F F V V V V V date P. A: ________ R.D.A.: ________

Thursday 8 8 8 8 8 8 8 8

______ F F F F F V V V V V

date

P. A: ________ R.D.A.: ________

Friday 8 8 8 8 8 8 8 8

______ F F F F F V V V V V

date

P. A: ________ R.D.A.: ________

Saturday 8 8 8 8 8 8 8 8

______ F F F F F V V V V V

date

P. A: ________ R.D.A.: ________

Notes ________________________

____

____

____

____

Weekly Caloric Intake ______-______

Sunday 8 8 8 8 8 8 8 8 ______ F F F F F V V V V V date P. A: ________ R.D.A.: ________
Monday 8 8 8 8 8 8 8 8 ______ F F F F F V V V V V date P. A: ________ R.D.A.: ________
Tuesday 8 8 8 8 8 8 8 8 ______ F F F F F V V V V V date P. A: ________ R.D.A.: ________
Wednesday 8 8 8 8 8 8 8 8 ______ F F F F F V V V V V date P. A: ________ R.D.A.: ________

Thursday 8 8 8 8 8 8 8 8

______ F F F F F V V V V V

date

P. A: ________ R.D.A.: ________

Friday 8 8 8 8 8 8 8 8

______ F F F F F V V V V V

date

P. A: ________ R.D.A.: ________

Saturday 8 8 8 8 8 8 8 8

______ F F F F F V V V V V

date

P. A: ________ R.D.A.: ________

Notes ________________________

____

____

____

____

Monthly Physical Activity

Log for: ________________________________

Next to each day of the week, write the total number of minutes you engaged in physical activity that day.

1	2	3	4

5	6	7	8

9	10	11	12

13	14	15	16

17	18	19	20

21	22	23	24

25	26	27	28

29	30	31	

Monthly Total = ______________

Weekly Caloric Intake ______-______

Sunday 8 8 8 8 8 8 8 8 ______ F F F F F V V V V V date P. A: ________ R.D.A.: ________
Monday 8 8 8 8 8 8 8 8 ______ F F F F F V V V V V date P. A: ________ R.D.A.: ________
Tuesday 8 8 8 8 8 8 8 8 ______ F F F F F V V V V V date P. A: ________ R.D.A.: ________
Wednesday 8 8 8 8 8 8 8 8 ______ F F F F F V V V V V date P. A: ________ R.D.A.: ________

Thursday 8 8 8 8 8 8 8 8

______ F F F F F V V V V V

date

P. A: ________ R.D.A.: ________

Friday 8 8 8 8 8 8 8 8

______ F F F F F V V V V V

date

P. A: ________ R.D.A.: ________

Saturday 8 8 8 8 8 8 8 8

______ F F F F F V V V V V

date

P. A: ________ R.D.A.: ________

Notes ________________________

Weekly Caloric Intake ______-______

Sunday 8 8 8 8 8 8 8 8 ______ F F F F F V V V V V date P. A: ________ R.D.A.: ________
Monday 8 8 8 8 8 8 8 8 ______ F F F F F V V V V V date P. A: ________ R.D.A.: ________
Tuesday 8 8 8 8 8 8 8 8 ______ F F F F F V V V V V date P. A: ________ R.D.A.: ________
Wednesday 8 8 8 8 8 8 8 8 ______ F F F F F V V V V V date P. A: ________ R.D.A.: ________

Thursday 8 8 8 8 8 8 8 8

______ F F F F F V V V V V

date

P. A: ________ R.D.A.: ________

Friday 8 8 8 8 8 8 8 8

______ F F F F F V V V V V

date

P. A: ________ R.D.A.: ________

Saturday 8 8 8 8 8 8 8 8

______ F F F F F V V V V V

date

P. A: ________ R.D.A.: ________

Notes ________________________

____

____

____

____

Weekly Caloric Intake ______-______

Sunday	8 8 8 8 8 8 8 8
______	F F F F F V V V V V
date	
P. A: ________	R.D.A.: ________
Monday	8 8 8 8 8 8 8 8
______	F F F F F V V V V V
date	
P. A: ________	R.D.A.: ________
Tuesday	8 8 8 8 8 8 8 8
______	F F F F F V V V V V
date	
P. A: ________	R.D.A.: ________
Wednesday	8 8 8 8 8 8 8 8
______	F F F F F V V V V V
date	
P. A: ________	R.D.A.: ________

Thursday 8 8 8 8 8 8 8 8

______ F F F F F V V V V V

date

P. A: ________ R.D.A.: ________

Friday 8 8 8 8 8 8 8 8

______ F F F F F V V V V V

date

P. A: ________ R.D.A.: ________

Saturday 8 8 8 8 8 8 8 8

______ F F F F F V V V V V

date

P. A: ________ R.D.A.: ________

Notes ______________________________

____

____

____

____

Weekly Caloric Intake ______-______

Sunday 8 8 8 8 8 8 8 8 ______ F F F F F V V V V V date P. A: ________ R.D.A.: ________
Monday 8 8 8 8 8 8 8 8 ______ F F F F F V V V V V date P. A: ________ R.D.A.: ________
Tuesday 8 8 8 8 8 8 8 8 ______ F F F F F V V V V V date P. A: ________ R.D.A.: ________
Wednesday 8 8 8 8 8 8 8 8 ______ F F F F F V V V V V date P. A: ________ R.D.A.: ________

Thursday 8 8 8 8 8 8 8 8

______ F F F F F V V V V V

date

P. A: ________ R.D.A.: ________

Friday 8 8 8 8 8 8 8 8

______ F F F F F V V V V V

date

P. A: ________ R.D.A.: ________

Saturday 8 8 8 8 8 8 8 8

______ F F F F F V V V V V

date

P. A: ________ R.D.A.: ________

Notes ________________________

____

____

____

____

Monthly Physical Activity

Log for: ______________________________

Next to each day of the week, write the total number of minutes you engaged in physical activity that day.

1	2	3	4

5	6	7	8

9	10	11	12

13	14	15	16

17	18	19	20

21	22	23	24

25	26	27	28

29	30	31	

Monthly Total = ________________

Weekly Caloric Intake _____-_____

Sunday 8 8 8 8 8 8 8 8 _____ F F F F F V V V V V date P. A: _______ R.D.A.: _______
Monday 8 8 8 8 8 8 8 8 _____ F F F F F V V V V V date P. A: _______ R.D.A.: _______
Tuesday 8 8 8 8 8 8 8 8 _____ F F F F F V V V V V date P. A: _______ R.D.A.: _______
Wednesday 8 8 8 8 8 8 8 8 _____ F F F F F V V V V V date P. A: _______ R.D.A.: _______

Thursday 8 8 8 8 8 8 8 8

______ F F F F F V V V V V

date

P. A: ________ R.D.A.: ________

Friday 8 8 8 8 8 8 8 8

______ F F F F F V V V V V

date

P. A: ________ R.D.A.: ________

Saturday 8 8 8 8 8 8 8 8

______ F F F F F V V V V V

date

P. A: ________ R.D.A.: ________

Notes ________________________

Weekly Caloric Intake _____-_____

Sunday 8 8 8 8 8 8 8 8 _____ F F F F F V V V V V date P. A: ________ R.D.A.: ________
Monday 8 8 8 8 8 8 8 8 _____ F F F F F V V V V V date P. A: ________ R.D.A.: ________
Tuesday 8 8 8 8 8 8 8 8 _____ F F F F F V V V V V date P. A: ________ R.D.A.: ________
Wednesday 8 8 8 8 8 8 8 8 _____ F F F F F V V V V V date P. A: ________ R.D.A.: ________

Thursday 8 8 8 8 8 8 8 8

______ F F F F F V V V V V

date

P. A: ________ R.D.A.: ________

Friday 8 8 8 8 8 8 8 8

______ F F F F F V V V V V

date

P. A: ________ R.D.A.: ________

Saturday 8 8 8 8 8 8 8 8

______ F F F F F V V V V V

date

P. A: ________ R.D.A.: ________

Notes ________________________

____

____

____

____

Weekly Caloric Intake ______-______

Sunday 8 8 8 8 8 8 8 8 ______ F F F F F V V V V V date P. A: ________ R.D.A.: ________
Monday 8 8 8 8 8 8 8 8 ______ F F F F F V V V V V date P. A: ________ R.D.A.: ________
Tuesday 8 8 8 8 8 8 8 8 ______ F F F F F V V V V V date P. A: ________ R.D.A.: ________
Wednesday 8 8 8 8 8 8 8 8 ______ F F F F F V V V V V date P. A: ________ R.D.A.: ________

Thursday 8 8 8 8 8 8 8 8

_____ F F F F F V V V V V

date

P. A: ________ R.D.A.: ________

Friday 8 8 8 8 8 8 8 8

_____ F F F F F V V V V V

date

P. A: ________ R.D.A.: ________

Saturday 8 8 8 8 8 8 8 8

_____ F F F F F V V V V V

date

P. A: ________ R.D.A.: ________

Notes ________________________

____

____

____

____

Weekly Caloric Intake _____-_____

Sunday 8 8 8 8 8 8 8 8

_____ F F F F F V V V V V

date

P. A: ________ R.D.A.: ________

Monday 8 8 8 8 8 8 8 8

_____ F F F F F V V V V V

date

P. A: ________ R.D.A.: ________

Tuesday 8 8 8 8 8 8 8 8

_____ F F F F F V V V V V

date

P. A: ________ R.D.A.: ________

Wednesday 8 8 8 8 8 8 8 8

_____ F F F F F V V V V V

date

P. A: ________ R.D.A.: ________

Thursday	8 8 8 8 8 8 8 8
_____ date	F F F F F V V V V V
P. A: ________	R.D.A.: ________
Friday	8 8 8 8 8 8 8 8
_____ date	F F F F F V V V V V
P. A: ________	R.D.A.: ________
Saturday	8 8 8 8 8 8 8 8
_____ date	F F F F F V V V V V
P. A: ________	R.D.A.: ________

Notes ______________________________

____

____

____

____

Monthly Physical Activity

Log for: ______________________________

Next to each day of the week, write the total number of minutes you engaged in physical activity that day.

1	2	3	4

5	6	7	8

9	10	11	12

13	14	15	16

17	18	19	20

21	22	23	24

25	26	27	28

29	30	31	

Monthly Total = ________________

Weekly Caloric Intake ______-______

Sunday 8 8 8 8 8 8 8 8 ______ F F F F F V V V V V date P. A: ________ R.D.A.: ________
Monday 8 8 8 8 8 8 8 8 ______ F F F F F V V V V V date P. A: ________ R.D.A.: ________
Tuesday 8 8 8 8 8 8 8 8 ______ F F F F F V V V V V date P. A: ________ R.D.A.: ________
Wednesday 8 8 8 8 8 8 8 8 ______ F F F F F V V V V V date P. A: ________ R.D.A.: ________

Thursday 8 8 8 8 8 8 8 8

______ F F F F F V V V V V

date

P. A: ________ R.D.A.: ________

Friday 8 8 8 8 8 8 8 8

______ F F F F F V V V V V

date

P. A: ________ R.D.A.: ________

Saturday 8 8 8 8 8 8 8 8

______ F F F F F V V V V V

date

P. A: ________ R.D.A.: ________

Notes ________________________

____

____

____

____

Section 6

Dates

________ to ________

Goals on Your Healthy for Life Journey

Goals

Check the box when a goal is achieved, and write the date it was achieved on the line next to the box. Write a goal next to the number, keeping in mind the ABCs.

Date Achieved | Goal

☐ ______ 1. ________________________________

☐ ______ 2. ________________________________

☐ ______ 3. ________________________________

☐ ______ 4. ________________________________

Measurement of *You* on Your Healthy for Life Journey

Date: ____________________

Location	Measurement
Neck	
Chest	
Bicep	
Waist	
Hips	
Thighs	
Weight	
BMI	

Picture of *You* on Your Healthy for Life Journey

Date: ______________________

Diabetes

Due to increases in childhood obesity across America, the number of children diagnosed with diabetes has drastically increased. This is a disease once seen only in adults, but today, type 2 diabetes is affecting more and more young children (CDC, 2011). In addition, diabetes is the seventh-leading cause of death nationally, with death tolls even higher among some ethnic groups. The distressing fact is that *type 2 diabetes is a disease that is almost entirely preventable with a balanced diet and exercise.* It is not an easy disease to manage in adulthood, much less for a child to have to deal with.

In May 2010, the White House Task Force on Childhood Obesity wrote a report to the president titled "Solving the Problem of Childhood Obesity within a Generation." The report stated that *one-third of all children born in the year 2000 and after are expected to develop diabetes.*

So what is diabetes? According to the CDC (2011), diabetes is a group of diseases marked by high levels of blood glucose that result from defects in insulin production, insulin action, or both. In addition, prediabetes is a condition similar to diabetes where individuals have higher-than-normal blood glucose levels, but the levels are not high enough to be classified as diabetes. However, people with prediabetes *are at risk of developing type 2 diabetes as well as heart disease and stroke*. Yet, studies have shown prediabetics who balance their scales or lose weight and increase their physical activity can prevent or delay type 2 diabetes, with some patients returning their blood glucose levels to normal.

There are four types of diabetes: type 1, type 2, gestational (seen during pregnancy), and other types, which include "specific genetic conditions (such as maturity-onset diabetes of youth, surgery, medications, infections, pancreatic disease, and other illnesses). Keep in mind other types of diabetes account for merely 1-5% of all diagnosed cases, with type 2 being the most prevalent in adults. In the United States, diabetes affects 25.8 million people of all ages, 18.8 million diagnosed and 7.0 million undiagnosed. In addition, it is estimated that 79 million Americans aged twenty and older have prediabetes.

In 2010, roughly a quarter of a million American people younger than twenty had either type 1 or type 2 diabetes, as well as 10.9 million people aged sixty-five and older. About 1.9 million people aged twenty or older were newly diagnosed. In addition to being the seventh-leading cause of death in the United States, diabetes is a major cause of heart disease and stroke, the leading cause of kidney failure, non-traumatic lower-limb amputations, and new cases of blindness among adults.

According to the CDC, overall, the risk of death among people with diabetes is about twice that of people of similar age who do not have diabetes. Complications of diabetes in the United States include:

- Heart disease and stroke
- Hypertension
- Blindness and eye problems
- Kidney disease
- Nervous system disease
- Amputations
- Dental disease
- Complications of pregnancy
- Biochemical imbalances

- More susceptible to many other illnesses
- Decreased mobility
- Depression

Lifestyle changes, including weight loss and increasing physical activity, have shown to reduce the development of type 2 diabetes and prediabetes.

Recommended Daily Allowance

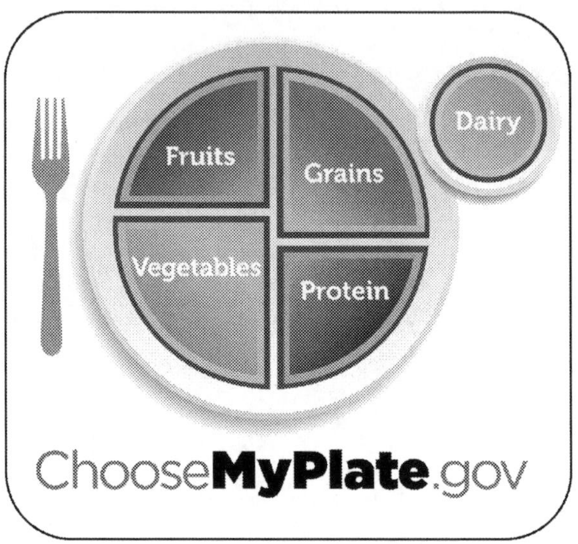

Go to the following website: www.choosemyplate.gov to find out what your recommend daily allowance (RDA), or caloric intake, should include and write it down.

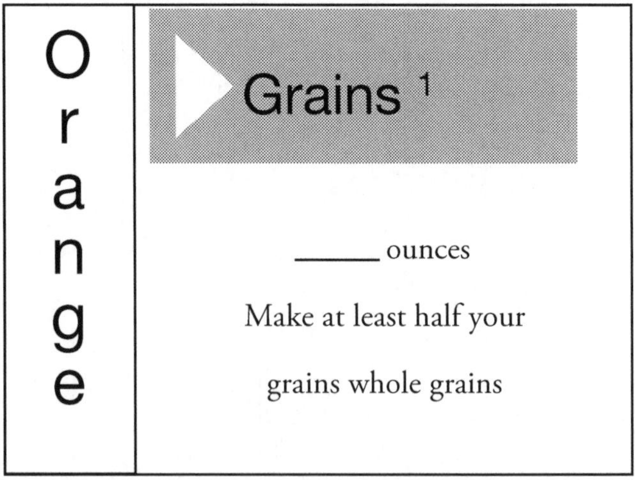

Green	**Vegetables** [2] _____ cups Try to include: dark green, red, & orange; beans & peas, starchy, & other veggies
Red	**Fruits** _____ cups Select fresh, frozen, canned, & dried fruit more often than juie
Blue	**Dairy** _____ cups Include fat-free and low-fat dairy foods every day

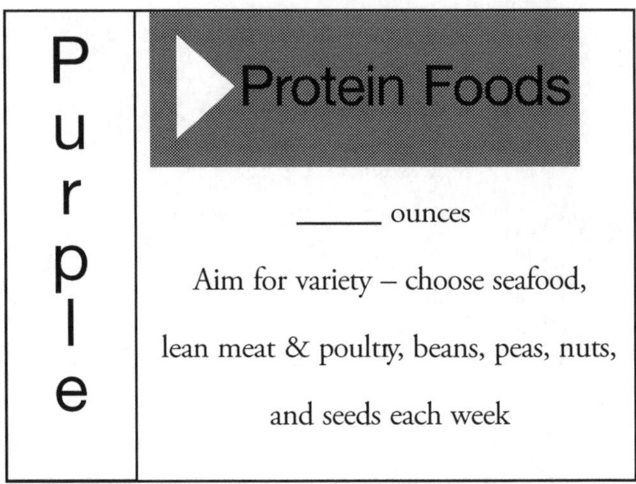

In a few months, go back to see if this has changed. As you begin to include more physical activity and your weight decreases to a healthier weight, these numbers may change.

Weekly Calorie Intake

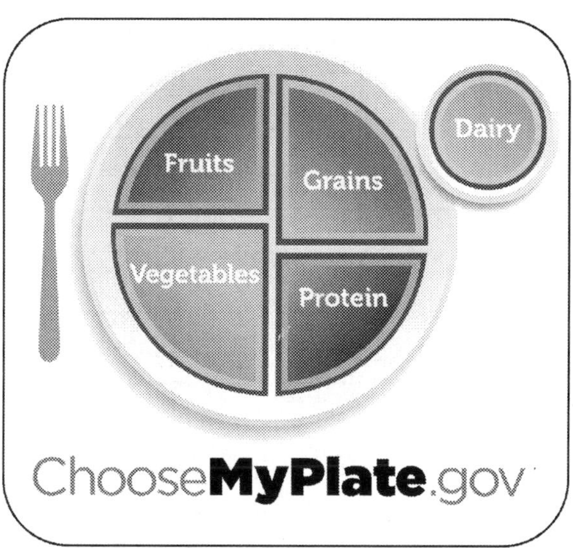

Weekly include:

Dark Green Vegetables: ______ cups

Orange Vegetables: ______ cups

Dry Beans & Peas: ______ cups

Starchy Vegetables: ______ cups

Other Vegetables: ______ cups

New Foods I will try this quarter

Grains: ______________________ __________________________ __________________________
Vegetables: ____________________ __________________________ __________________________
Fruits: _______________________ __________________________ __________________________
Dairy: _______________________ __________________________ __________________________
Protein: ______________________ __________________________ __________________________

How to use your weekly caloric intake log:

Write the date under the day of the week.

8: cross off an 8 for each eight ounces of water you drink each day.

F: cross off an F for each fruit you eat each day.

V: cross off a V for each vegetable you eat each day.

P.A.: write the number of minutes you participated in physical activity each day.

RDA: write a Y or N if you kept within your RDA.

There should be enough for each section, which includes three months each.

Journal Entries

Weekly Caloric Intake ______-______

Sunday 8 8 8 8 8 8 8 8 ______ F F F F F V V V V V date P. A: ________ R.D.A.: ________
Monday 8 8 8 8 8 8 8 8 ______ F F F F F V V V V V date P. A: ________ R.D.A.: ________
Tuesday 8 8 8 8 8 8 8 8 ______ F F F F F V V V V V date P. A: ________ R.D.A.: ________
Wednesday 8 8 8 8 8 8 8 8 ______ F F F F F V V V V V date P. A: ________ R.D.A.: ________

Thursday 8 8 8 8 8 8 8 8 ______ F F F F F V V V V V date P. A: ________ R.D.A.: ________
Friday 8 8 8 8 8 8 8 8 ______ F F F F F V V V V V date P. A: ________ R.D.A.: ________
Saturday 8 8 8 8 8 8 8 8 ______ F F F F F V V V V V date P. A: ________ R.D.A.: ________
Notes ____________________ ________________________ ________________________ ________________________ ________________________

Weekly Caloric Intake ______-______

Sunday 8 8 8 8 8 8 8 8
______ F F F F F V V V V V
date
P. A: ________ R.D.A.: ________
Monday 8 8 8 8 8 8 8 8
______ F F F F F V V V V V
date
P. A: ________ R.D.A.: ________
Tuesday 8 8 8 8 8 8 8 8
______ F F F F F V V V V V
date
P. A: ________ R.D.A.: ________
Wednesday 8 8 8 8 8 8 8 8
______ F F F F F V V V V V
date
P. A: ________ R.D.A.: ________

Thursday 8 8 8 8 8 8 8 8

_____ F F F F F V V V V V

date

P. A: ________ R.D.A.: ________

Friday 8 8 8 8 8 8 8 8

_____ F F F F F V V V V V

date

P. A: ________ R.D.A.: ________

Saturday 8 8 8 8 8 8 8 8

_____ F F F F F V V V V V

date

P. A: ________ R.D.A.: ________

Notes ________________________

____

____

____

____

Weekly Caloric Intake ______-______

Sunday 8 8 8 8 8 8 8 8 ______ F F F F F V V V V V date P. A: ________ R.D.A.: ________
Monday 8 8 8 8 8 8 8 8 ______ F F F F F V V V V V date P. A: ________ R.D.A.: ________
Tuesday 8 8 8 8 8 8 8 8 ______ F F F F F V V V V V date P. A: ________ R.D.A.: ________
Wednesday 8 8 8 8 8 8 8 8 ______ F F F F F V V V V V date P. A: ________ R.D.A.: ________

Thursday 8 8 8 8 8 8 8 8

______ F F F F F V V V V V

date

P. A: ________ R.D.A.: ________

Friday 8 8 8 8 8 8 8 8

______ F F F F F V V V V V

date

P. A: ________ R.D.A.: ________

Saturday 8 8 8 8 8 8 8 8

______ F F F F F V V V V V

date

P. A: ________ R.D.A.: ________

Notes ________________________

____

____

____

____

Weekly Caloric Intake _____-_____

Sunday 8 8 8 8 8 8 8 8 _____ F F F F F V V V V V date P. A: ________ R.D.A.: ________
Monday 8 8 8 8 8 8 8 8 _____ F F F F F V V V V V date P. A: ________ R.D.A.: ________
Tuesday 8 8 8 8 8 8 8 8 _____ F F F F F V V V V V date P. A: ________ R.D.A.: ________
Wednesday 8 8 8 8 8 8 8 8 _____ F F F F F V V V V V date P. A: ________ R.D.A.: ________

Thursday 8 8 8 8 8 8 8 8

______ F F F F F V V V V V

date

P. A: ________ R.D.A.: ________

Friday 8 8 8 8 8 8 8 8

______ F F F F F V V V V V

date

P. A: ________ R.D.A.: ________

Saturday 8 8 8 8 8 8 8 8

______ F F F F F V V V V V

date

P. A: ________ R.D.A.: ________

Notes ________________________

Monthly Physical Activity

Log for: ______________________________

Next to each day of the week, write the total number of minutes you engaged in physical activity that day.

1	2	3	4

5	6	7	8

9	10	11	12

13	14	15	16

17	18	19	20

21	22	23	24

25	26	27	28

29	30	31	

Monthly Total = ______________

Weekly Caloric Intake ______-______

Sunday 8 8 8 8 8 8 8 8

______ F F F F F V V V V V

date

P. A: ________ R.D.A.: ________

Monday 8 8 8 8 8 8 8 8

______ F F F F F V V V V V

date

P. A: ________ R.D.A.: ________

Tuesday 8 8 8 8 8 8 8 8

______ F F F F F V V V V V

date

P. A: ________ R.D.A.: ________

Wednesday 8 8 8 8 8 8 8 8

______ F F F F F V V V V V

date

P. A: ________ R.D.A.: ________

Thursday 8 8 8 8 8 8 8 8

_____ F F F F F V V V V V

date

P. A: ________ R.D.A.: ________

Friday 8 8 8 8 8 8 8 8

_____ F F F F F V V V V V

date

P. A: ________ R.D.A.: ________

Saturday 8 8 8 8 8 8 8 8

_____ F F F F F V V V V V

date

P. A: ________ R.D.A.: ________

Notes ________________________

____

____

____

____

Weekly Caloric Intake ______-______

Sunday 8 8 8 8 8 8 8 8 ______ F F F F F V V V V V date P. A: ________ R.D.A.: ________
Monday 8 8 8 8 8 8 8 8 ______ F F F F F V V V V V date P. A: ________ R.D.A.: ________
Tuesday 8 8 8 8 8 8 8 8 ______ F F F F F V V V V V date P. A: ________ R.D.A.: ________
Wednesday 8 8 8 8 8 8 8 8 ______ F F F F F V V V V V date P. A: ________ R.D.A.: ________

Thursday 8 8 8 8 8 8 8 8

_____ F F F F F V V V V V

date

P. A: ________ R.D.A.: ________

Friday 8 8 8 8 8 8 8 8

_____ F F F F F V V V V V

date

P. A: ________ R.D.A.: ________

Saturday 8 8 8 8 8 8 8 8

_____ F F F F F V V V V V

date

P. A: ________ R.D.A.: ________

Notes ________________________

____

____

____

____

Weekly Caloric Intake ______-______

Sunday 8 8 8 8 8 8 8 8

______ F F F F F V V V V V

date

P. A: ________ R.D.A.: ________

Monday 8 8 8 8 8 8 8 8

______ F F F F F V V V V V

date

P. A: ________ R.D.A.: ________

Tuesday 8 8 8 8 8 8 8 8

______ F F F F F V V V V V

date

P. A: ________ R.D.A.: ________

Wednesday 8 8 8 8 8 8 8 8

______ F F F F F V V V V V

date

P. A: ________ R.D.A.: ________

Thursday 88888888

______ FFFFF VVVVV

date

P. A: ________ R.D.A.: ________

Friday 88888888

______ FFFFF VVVVV

date

P. A: ________ R.D.A.: ________

Saturday 88888888

______ FFFFF VVVVV

date

P. A: ________ R.D.A.: ________

Notes ________________________

____

____

____

____

Weekly Caloric Intake ______-______

Sunday 8 8 8 8 8 8 8 8 ______ F F F F F V V V V V date P. A: ________ R.D.A.: ________
Monday 8 8 8 8 8 8 8 8 ______ F F F F F V V V V V date P. A: ________ R.D.A.: ________
Tuesday 8 8 8 8 8 8 8 8 ______ F F F F F V V V V V date P. A: ________ R.D.A.: ________
Wednesday 8 8 8 8 8 8 8 8 ______ F F F F F V V V V V date P. A: ________ R.D.A.: ________

Thursday 8 8 8 8 8 8 8 8

______ F F F F F V V V V V

date

P. A: ________ R.D.A.: ________

Friday 8 8 8 8 8 8 8 8

______ F F F F F V V V V V

date

P. A: ________ R.D.A.: ________

Saturday 8 8 8 8 8 8 8 8

______ F F F F F V V V V V

date

P. A: ________ R.D.A.: ________

Notes ________________________

____

____

____

____

Monthly Physical Activity

Log for: ______________________________

Next to each day of the week, write the total number of minutes you engaged in physical activity that day.

1	2	3	4

5	6	7	8

9	10	11	12

13	14	15	16

17	18	19	20

21	22	23	24

25	26	27	28

29	30	31	

Monthly Total = ______________

Weekly Caloric Intake _____-_____

Sunday 8 8 8 8 8 8 8 8 _____ F F F F F V V V V V date P. A: ________ R.D.A.: ________
Monday 8 8 8 8 8 8 8 8 _____ F F F F F V V V V V date P. A: ________ R.D.A.: ________
Tuesday 8 8 8 8 8 8 8 8 _____ F F F F F V V V V V date P. A: ________ R.D.A.: ________
Wednesday 8 8 8 8 8 8 8 8 _____ F F F F F V V V V V date P. A: ________ R.D.A.: ________

Thursday 8 8 8 8 8 8 8 8

______ F F F F F V V V V V

date

P. A: ________ R.D.A.: ________

Friday 8 8 8 8 8 8 8 8

______ F F F F F V V V V V

date

P. A: ________ R.D.A.: ________

Saturday 8 8 8 8 8 8 8 8

______ F F F F F V V V V V

date

P. A: ________ R.D.A.: ________

Notes ________________________

____

____

____

____

Weekly Caloric Intake ______-______

Sunday	8 8 8 8 8 8 8 8
______ date	F F F F F V V V V V
P. A: __________	R.D.A.: __________
Monday	8 8 8 8 8 8 8 8
______ date	F F F F F V V V V V
P. A: __________	R.D.A.: __________
Tuesday	8 8 8 8 8 8 8 8
______ date	F F F F F V V V V V
P. A: __________	R.D.A.: __________
Wednesday	8 8 8 8 8 8 8 8
______ date	F F F F F V V V V V
P. A: __________	R.D.A.: __________

Thursday 8 8 8 8 8 8 8 8

______ F F F F F V V V V V

date

P. A: ________ R.D.A.: ________

Friday 8 8 8 8 8 8 8 8

______ F F F F F V V V V V

date

P. A: ________ R.D.A.: ________

Saturday 8 8 8 8 8 8 8 8

______ F F F F F V V V V V

date

P. A: ________ R.D.A.: ________

Notes ________________________

____

____

____

____

Weekly Caloric Intake _____-_____

Sunday 8 8 8 8 8 8 8 8 _____ F F F F F V V V V V date P. A: ________ R.D.A.: ________
Monday 8 8 8 8 8 8 8 8 _____ F F F F F V V V V V date P. A: ________ R.D.A.: ________
Tuesday 8 8 8 8 8 8 8 8 _____ F F F F F V V V V V date P. A: ________ R.D.A.: ________
Wednesday 8 8 8 8 8 8 8 8 _____ F F F F F V V V V V date P. A: ________ R.D.A.: ________

Thursday 8 8 8 8 8 8 8 8

______ F F F F F V V V V V

date

P. A: ________ R.D.A.: ________

Friday 8 8 8 8 8 8 8 8

______ F F F F F V V V V V

date

P. A: ________ R.D.A.: ________

Saturday 8 8 8 8 8 8 8 8

______ F F F F F V V V V V

date

P. A: ________ R.D.A.: ________

Notes ________________________

____

____

____

____

Weekly Caloric Intake _____-_____

Sunday 8 8 8 8 8 8 8 8 _____ F F F F F V V V V V date P. A: _______ R.D.A.: _______
Monday 8 8 8 8 8 8 8 8 _____ F F F F F V V V V V date P. A: _______ R.D.A.: _______
Tuesday 8 8 8 8 8 8 8 8 _____ F F F F F V V V V V date P. A: _______ R.D.A.: _______
Wednesday 8 8 8 8 8 8 8 8 _____ F F F F F V V V V V date P. A: _______ R.D.A.: _______

Thursday 8 8 8 8 8 8 8 8

_____ F F F F F V V V V V

date

P. A: ________ R.D.A.: ________

Friday 8 8 8 8 8 8 8 8

_____ F F F F F V V V V V

date

P. A: ________ R.D.A.: ________

Saturday 8 8 8 8 8 8 8 8

_____ F F F F F V V V V V

date

P. A: ________ R.D.A.: ________

Notes ____________________

Monthly Physical Activity

Log for: ______________________________

Next to each day of the week, write the total number of minutes you engaged in physical activity that day.

1	2	3	4

5	6	7	8

9	10	11	12

13	14	15	16

17	18	19	20

21	22	23	24

25	26	27	28

29	30	31	

Monthly Total = ______________

Weekly Caloric Intake ______-______

Sunday 8 8 8 8 8 8 8 8 ______ F F F F F V V V V V date P. A: ________ R.D.A.: ________
Monday 8 8 8 8 8 8 8 8 ______ F F F F F V V V V V date P. A: ________ R.D.A.: ________
Tuesday 8 8 8 8 8 8 8 8 ______ F F F F F V V V V V date P. A: ________ R.D.A.: ________
Wednesday 8 8 8 8 8 8 8 8 ______ F F F F F V V V V V date P. A: ________ R.D.A.: ________

Thursday 8 8 8 8 8 8 8 8

_____ F F F F F V V V V V

date

P. A: ________ R.D.A.: ________

Friday 8 8 8 8 8 8 8 8

_____ F F F F F V V V V V

date

P. A: ________ R.D.A.: ________

Saturday 8 8 8 8 8 8 8 8

_____ F F F F F V V V V V

date

P. A: ________ R.D.A.: ________

Notes ________________________

____

____

____

____

Keep Your Scale Balanced

I hope this journal provides you with the tools you need to help you live a healthy for life lifestyle. More than anything, I hope you do not become a statistic of childhood obesity and that you, your family, your friends, and even those who are not even in your life yet will benefit from your healthy for life lifestyle.

I know there will be times when you want to indulge in a plate full of unhealthy, great-tasting foods. However, I hope you plan for that plate full of unhealthy, great-tasting foods or balance your scale with sufficient physical activity.

I remember when I finally reached a healthy weight; it was the week before my birthday. My girlfriends, Erlinda and Gerri, took me out to eat. Our tradition is on each of our birthdays, we eat dessert first! Later that week, my parents, my family, and my husband had a surprise birthday party for me. Also, my students decorated my door and my office, and I had even more cake! By the time my birthday celebrations were finally over, my healthy weight was teetering, and I was going backward.

When the parties finally ended, the first thing I did was increase my physical activity and decrease my caloric intake. Before long, I was once again balanced and at a healthy weight. Stay accountable to yourself, and always be honest! And *never, ever* jump and run from the balance of being healthy for life.

A Final Word

Today I actually received word my book, *It's Not About Childhood Obesity, It Is about Being Healthy for Life,* had been moved into production—a day I have been waiting for impatiently for some time. Tomorrow is Halloween.

When I picked up my children—ages four, six, and seven—they were all speaking simultaneously about the parties in class tomorrow as we walked through the rain; I was on crutches.

Then my daughter began her speech to me, something like this (yes, it went on forever): "Now Mom, tomorrow we are having parties in class, but my teacher said we have to bring individually wrapped food, and Mom, we cannot just take a bunch of candy and junk food, we have to take healthy food too because just because it's Halloween does not mean we just eat junk ,and that is not healthy anyway, so when you make our snacks, Mom, you better not just be making junk because that is bad and not good for us and we need to be healthy and that helps us learn better, okay, Mom!"

That night we celebrated my book, and my daughter said, "Congratulations on your book, Mom!" To me, the irony of the evening was she was congratulating me on a book I wrote about childhood obesity, yet she gave *me* a speech that lasted forever about how I better not just make a bunch of junk because it was Halloween. I knew then if I had not made a positive difference in what she eats, maybe her teacher might, and she just might live healthy for life!

Good luck, *God's* blessing, and keep your scale balanced!

About the Author

Dr. Olga Vaca Durr worked in the education field for fourteen years, in both elementary and secondary education, as well as in school and district administration. She has degrees in elementary and special education, educational administration, and a doctorate in educational leadership, with specializations in early childhood, bilingual education, and educational diagnostics. She is currently working on a book for parents and adults, also about childhood obesity. Olga finds herself juggling the arduous tasks of being a military wife, mother of three young, very active children, and her journey toward being healthy for life. Olga, her husband, and her children call Texas home. However, the military takes them on many adventures.

Glossary

Body mass index (BMI): a reliable indicator of body fatness for most children and teens. It is calculated according to a child's weight and height and is age- and sex-specific for children and teens. The formula for adults to calculate BMI is as follows: weight (pounds)/height (inches) 2 x 703.

Caloric intake: calories that are consumed.

Exercise: a subset of physical activity that is planned, structured, and repetitive. Its purpose is to improve or maintain physical fitness.

Globesity: the global epidemic of obesity or how obesity is affecting so many countries throughout the world.

Kinesiology: the study of the mechanics of body movements.

Obesity: a term the Centers for Disease Control stated is two categories above a healthy weight range and includes a body mass index (BMI) of 30 or more.

Physical activity: bodily motion resulting in energy expenditure that is produced by skeletal muscles.

Physical fitness: a subset of exercises that are either health- or skill-related.

Portion size: how much you choose to eat during either a meal or snack, so a portion is as big or as small as you want it to be.

Sedentary activities: activities involving sitting and correspondingly little motion or exercise.

Serving size: a fixed amount of food, such as one cup or one ounce, shown on the nutrition facts label. It is useful in determining how much of that particular food you eat and what amount of nutrients you are getting, and in making comparisons among foods.

Resources

American Cancer Society

http://www.cancer.org/

American Diabetes Services

http://www.americandiabetes.com/

American Heart Association

http://www.heart.org/HEARTORG/

"Be Active, Healthy, and Happy!" 2008 Physical Activity Guidelines for Americans by the US Department of Health and Human Services

http://www.health.gov/paguidelines/guidelines/default.aspx

BMI Percentile Calculator for Child and Teen, Centers for Disease Control and Prevention

http://apps.nccd.cdc.gov/dnpabmi/

Centers for Disease Control and Prevention

http://www.cdc.gov/

Centers for Disease Control and Prevention, Fruits and Veggies More Matters

http://www.fruitsandveggiesmatter.gov/

Cooper Institute, The

http://www.cooperinstitute.org/

Dietary Guidelines for Americans 2010, booklet, by US Department of Agriculture and US Department of Health and Human Services

http://health.gov/dietaryguidelines/dga2010/DietaryGuidelines2010.pdf

Fitnessgram

http://www.fitnessgram.net/home/

Kids' Health

http://kidshealth.org/kid/

Let's Move, America's Move to Raise a Healthier Generation of Kids

http://www.letsmove.gov/

Media-Smart Youth: Eat, Think, and Be Active. National Institutes of Health, Eunice Kennedy Shriver, National Institute of Child Health and Human Development

http://www.nichd.nih.gov/msy/

National Cancer Institute at the National Institutes of Health

http://www.cancer.gov/

National Football League, Play 60

http://www.nfl.com/play60

National Institutes of Health, Eunice Kennedy Shriver, National Institute of Child Health & Human Development

http://www.nichd.nih.gov/milk/milk.cfm

Navy Operational Fueling, by the US Department of the Navy

http://www.cnrc.navy.mil/noru/html/downloads/NOFFS_Nutrition.pdf

President's Challenge, The

https://www.presidentschallenge.org/

"Take Charge of Your Health," by US Department of Health and Human Services

http://win.niddk.nih.gov/publications/PDFs/teenblackwhite3.pdf

Trust for America's Health, Preventing Epidemics, Protecting People

http://healthyamericans.org/

US Department of Agriculture, Centers for Nutrition Policy and Promotion

http://www.cnpp.usda.gov/

US Department of Agriculture, Food, and Nutrition Service website

http://teamnutrition.usda.gov/Default.htm

US Department of Agriculture, Know Your Farmer, Know Your Food

http://www.usda.gov/wps/portal/usda/knowyourfarmer?navid=KNOWYOURFARMER

US Department of Agriculture, My Plate.gov

http://www.choosemyplate.gov/

US Department of Agriculture, The People's Garden

http://www.usda.gov/wps/portal/usda/usdahome?navid=PEOPLES_GARDEN

US Department of Health and Human Services

http://www.nih.gov/

US Department of Health and Human Services, "Deliciously Healthy Eating" (includes various healthy eating recipes)

http://hp2010.nhlbihin.net/healthyeating/default.aspx

US Department of Health and Human Services, National Institute of Diabetes and Digestive and Kidney Diseases

http://www2.niddk.nih.gov/

US Department of Health and Human Services, US Food and Drug Administration

http://www.fda.gov/

References

Centers for Disease Control and Prevention (2011). *National diabetes fact sheet: national estimates and general information on diabetes and prediabetes in the United States, 2011.* Retrieved from http://www.cdc.gov/diabetes/pubs/pdf/ndfs_2011.pdf.

Centers for Disease Control and Prevention (2010). *Childhood overweight and obesity.* Retrieved from *http://www.cdc.gov/obesity/childhood/index.html.*

Schumacher, D., and Queen, J. A., *Overcoming Obesity in Childhood and Adolescence: A Guide for School Leaders.* Thousand Oaks, CA: Corwin Press, 2007.

US Department of Agriculture (1999). *Food portions and servings, how do they differ?* Retrieved from *http://www.cnpp.usda.gov/Publications/NutritionInsights/insight11.pdf.*

US Department of Health and Human Services, Centers for Disease Control and Prevention (2010). *Health, United States, 2010, with special feature on death and dying.* Retrieved from http://www.cdc.gov/nchs/data/hus/hus10.pdf.

US Department of Health and Human Services, National Institutes of Health (2009). *Portion Distortion*. Retrieved from *http://hp2010.nhlbihin.net/portion/index.htm.*

US Department of Health and Human Services (2008). *2008 Physical activity guidelines for Americans*. Retrieved from www.health.gov/paguidelines.

US Department of Health and Human Services, Centers for Disease Control Prevention (2007). *What is body mass index?* Retrieved from *http://www.cdc.gov/nccdphp/dnpa/bmi/adult_BMI/about_adult_BMI.htm.*

US Department of the Navy (2010). *Navy Operational Fueling*. Retrieved from *http://www.cnrc.navy.mil/noru/html/downloads/NOFFS_Nutrition.pdf.*

Vaca Durr, O. A. (2010). "The Relationship between Physical Fitness and Academic Achievement in Math and Science in a Select Texas School District." Unpublished doctoral dissertation, University of Mary Hardin Baylor, Belton, Texas.

Vaca Durr, O. A., *It's Not About Childhood Obesity, It IS About Being Healthy for Life*. Bloomfield, IN: Inspiring Voices, 2012.

White House Task Force on Childhood Obesity. (2010). *Solving the problem of childhood obesity within a generation, White House task force on childhood obesity report to the president*. Retrieved from *http://www.letsmove.gov/tfco_fullreport_may2010.pdf.*